DATE DUE

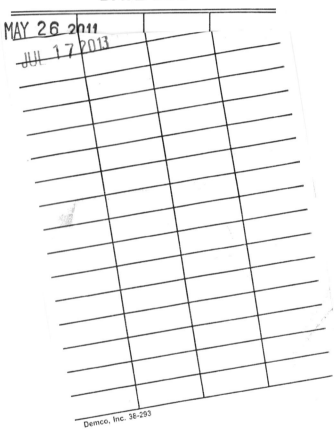

MAY 26 2011

JUL 17 2013

Military Life

Military Life is a series of books for service members and their families who must deal with the significant yet often overlooked difficulties unique to life in the military. Each of the titles in the series is a comprehensive presentation of the problems that arise, solutions to these problems, and resources that are of much further help. The authors of these books—who are themselves military members and experienced writers—have personally faced these challenging situations, and understand the many complications that accompany them. This is the first stop for members of the military and their loved ones in search of information on navigating the complex world of military life.

1. *The Wounded Warrior Handbook: A Resource Guide for Returning Veterans* by Don Philpott and Janelle Hill (2008).
2. *The Military Marriage Manual: Tactics for Successful Relationships* by Janelle Hill, Cheryl Lawhorne, and Don Philpott (2010).
3. *Combat-Related Traumatic Brain Injury and PTSD: A Resource and Recovery Guide* by Cheryl Lawhorne and Don Philpott (2010).
4. *Special Needs Families in the Military: A Resource Guide* by Janelle Hill and Don Philpott (2010).

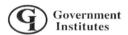 **Government Institutes**

Published by Government Institutes
An imprint of The Scarecrow Press, Inc.
A wholly owned subsidary of The Rowman & Littlefield Publishing Group, Inc.
4501 Forbes Boulevard, Suite 200, Lanham, Maryland 20706
http://www.govinstpress.com

Estover Road, Plymouth PL6 7PY, United Kingdom

British Library Cataloguing in Publication Information Available

Library of Congress Cataloging-in-Publication Data

Lawhorne, Cheryl, 1968-
   Combat-related traumatic brain injury and PTSD : a resource and recovery guide / Cheryl Lawhorne and Don Philpott.
      p.   ; cm.— (Military life ; 3)
   Includes bibliographical references and index.
   ISBN 978-1-60590-723-9 (cloth : alk. paper)—ISBN 978-1-60590-724-6 (electronic)
   1. Veterans—Mental health.   2. Post-traumatic stress disorder.   I. Philpott, Don, 1946–   II. Government Institutes.   III. Title.   IV. Series: Military life (Lanham, Md.) ; 3.
   [DNLM: 1. Combat Disorders.   2. Brain Injuries—complications.   3. Brain Injuries—psychology.   4. Stress Disorders, Post-Traumatic.   5. Veterans—psychology.   6. War. WM 184]
   RC550.L37   2010
   616.85'212—dc22
                                                                                      2010042118

♾ ™ The paper used in this publication meets the minimum requirements of American National Standard for Information Sciences—Permanence of Paper for Printed Library Materials, ANSI/NISO Z39.48-1992.

Printed in the United States of America

Contents

Foreword

I learned the hard way that the war doesn't stop when our boots touch home soil again; it just changes form.

Fighting my way free of PTSD's crippling effects took every reserve of strength I possessed. I could not have done it alone. Yet, as I traveled around the country, I met countless combat veterans who have never reached out, never sought the help they needed to cope with the trauma they experienced. We're tough guys, and tough guys don't need help. For generations, that's been the ethos in the military. And sure, we can survive and endure any manner of physical test—we're trained to do that. But none of us received any training on how to cope with the physiological changes acute trauma can cause in a human being.

I teamed up with John Bruning to write *Shadow of the Sword*, which chronicles my experiences in Fallujah as well as my struggle to conquer post-traumatic stress. The truth is, none of us who suffer from PTSD will ever be totally free of its symptoms. We have to learn to manage them, learn to recognize how they affect us, and develop coping skills to mitigate their effects. It is not an easy battle, but it is one that almost half of all soldiers and marines face as they return from Iraq and Afghanistan. Given the fluid nature of the fighting overseas right now, one expert has called the global war on terror the perfect incubator for PTSD.

This guidebook serves as a beacon to those who suffer behind closed doors as a way to let them know they are not the only ones going through this ordeal. They need to reach out and get help, because no man or woman can conquer this alone. Each soldier and marine we lose to suicide here in the states is a combat casualty, sure as anyone else who died in theater. The goal of the book is to destigmatize PTSD and show readers that courage and heroism on the battlefield comes with a heavy price. We are proud warriors and patriots, but here at home we need more than just parades and yellow ribbon magnets. We need support, help, and understanding.

In working with service members for over ten years, and writing on PTSD and traumatic brain injury, Cheryl Lawhorne and Don Philpott provide a much valued resource to all service members, their families, and the community. Her unwavering commitment to comprehensive care throughout all phases of recovery and long-term transition makes her a subject matter expert in the Wounded Warrior initiative.

Semper Fidelis.

Jeremiah Workman

Jeremiah Workman, SSgt USMC (ret.), currently works for the Wounded Warrior Regiment, HQMC, as the Civilian Deputy for the District Injured Support Cell. He is the author of *Shadow of the Sword* and was awarded the Navy Cross for gallantry under fire.

Preface

In 2009, more U.S. troops were hospitalized for mental health disorders than for battle wounds or other injuries—17,530 compared to 11,156, according to Pentagon statistics. A major reason was "the prolonged exposure to combat" as a result of multiple deployments during the last nine years of war.

Traumatic brain injury (TBI) is often referred to as the "signature wound" of the global war on terror. It's been reported that TBI could account for up to 50 percent of combat-related casualties and because of advances in trauma treatment, surgery, and rapid evacuation, many wounded warriors are now surviving what would just a few years ago have been fatal wounds. Many hundreds of thousands more service personnel are suffering from post-traumatic stress disorder (PTSD)—and, in many cases, don't realize it.

The purpose of this book is to look at TBI and PTSD—what they are; what are the treatment options; and what are the implications in terms of recovery, family relations, returning to service, or transitioning out and finding a job or going back to school, or requiring long-term care.

For wounded warriors with traumatic brain injury there are now excellent treatment facilities, such as the National Intrepid Center of Excellence on the Navy Campus at Bethesda, Maryland, next to the new Walter Reed National Military Medical Center. There is an ever growing network of support groups—both official and unofficial—and a dedicated army of caregivers.

It is fair to say that the consequences of PTSD weren't fully appreciated until quite recently. Many people believed it was simply the modern-day version of shell shock—you got it and you got over it.

Now, the physiological and psychological consequences are much better understood and the facilities that have been put in place are much better equipped at handling these problems. PTSD can manifest itself at any time.

U.S. WAR CASUALTIES

IRAQ DEATHS
Combat	3,492
Noncombat	928

IRAQ WOUNDED
Returned to duty	18,029
Not returned to duty within 72 hours	13,905

OPERATION NEW DAWN DEATHS
Combat	2
Noncombat	0

OPERATION NEW DAWN WOUNDED
Returned to duty	7
Not returned to duty within 72 hours	10

AFGHANISTAN DEATHS
Combat	970
Noncombat	298

AFGHANISTAN WOUNDED
Returned to duty	3,762
Not returned to duty within 72 hours	4,279

Source: DoD. www.defense.gov/news/casualty.pdf (as of September 14, 2010)

Many returning warriors don't realize they have PTSD but exhibit a wide range of other symptoms that suggest they do. Every day more and more facilities and support services are put in place to provide help to these wounded warriors and their loved ones.

While it is advanced technology that has contributed to the survival rate of these warriors, it is also advanced technology that can assist them in coping and dealing with their challenges. Above all, however, these wounded warriors, whether suffering from TBI or PTSD, need care and loving attention. Thankfully, there are many willing to give it and to all of them, our grateful and continuing thanks.

This book has been written as an easy-to-use reference guide for injured service members as well as for their families and loved ones. There is a huge and growing amount of literature available from the military and others; there are scores of support organizations involved in this arena and there are hundreds of websites offering information and help. All of these do a magnificent job in their respective areas, but it can be a daunting task to pull together all this information, especially at a time of crisis. The information in this book has been gathered from literally hundreds of these sources in the public domain.

A lot of the information included in this book comes from the Department of Veterans Affairs, the Department of Defense, and all branches of the services. We acknowledge their cooperation and have made every effort to be as up to date and accurate as possible.

Our aim is to provide a comprehensive framework that will allow you to quickly access information that you need regarding medical treatment, rehabilitation, counseling, support, transition, and if needed, long-term care. We also deal with financial, legal, and tax matters, although this book is a guide only and is not a legal, claims, or medical handbook. If you have detailed questions in these and other specialist areas you must seek the advice of an appropriate expert.

However, we hope that there is sufficient information to give you a better understanding of treatments, procedures, processes, and policies so that you know what is going on, what your rights are, and how you can benefit as a result.

Introduction

A History of Deployed Forces

TRENDS

The size and configuration of the U.S. military force have changed continuously throughout history, reflecting the defense needs of the country. Early in U.S. history, the concept of a standing army was less popular due to concerns about incurred costs and the fears of the impact of military power on the political process. The Second Continental Congress created the first regular active U.S. fighting force on June 14, 1775, and named it the Continental Army. Its purpose was to supplement local militia in fighting the British during the American Revolution. Upon the conclusion of that war the Continental Army was disbanded. Militia forces returned to their homes as well, available for call up only during times when national or state security required.

By early in the nineteenth century the need for a regular army was clear as militia forces could not be routinely relied upon for rapid and professional response to national crises. Since that time, the end strength of the Army has varied, typically rising during periods of war and decreasing during peacetime. The size of the combined U.S. Armed Forces reached an all-time high of 8.3 million during World War II. Through the Vietnam War, military members were conscripted in order to achieve necessary force strength. In 1973, at the end of the Vietnam War, the all-male draft that was initiated as the Selective Service Act of 1948 was terminated. Since that time the military has comprised an all-volunteer force. During the period of Operation Desert Storm, the U.S. Army totaled approximately 750,000 service members. This number decreased to its current number of just fewer than 500,000 personnel by the mid-1990s, its smallest size since the beginning of World War II.

Today the military has become a more diverse and complex population than ever in its history. Ethnic minorities make up significant portions of the armed forces, ranging from 24 percent in the Air Force to 40 percent in the Army (www.defense.gov/admin/about.html). Since the American Revolution, about 2 million women have served in the military. Today, about 16 percent of the active U.S. Armed Forces are women. In addition, over 50 percent of service members are married and about 11 percent of the marriages are to other service members. Although educational levels vary somewhat between branches of service, over 95 percent of the military has either a high school diploma or has passed the General Educational Development high school equivalency test. All four military branches have active as well as reserve components. Additionally, the Air Force and the Army also have National Guard components. These components are discussed below. As outlined in the Constitution, the U.S. Congress sets the end-strength for all services.

National Guard and Reserve Components

The National Guard was formed from the earlier state militias. Congress officially designated the National Guard in 1916, establishing procedures for training and equipping these units to active duty military standards. In so doing, the Congress made these state defense National Guard units available in times of national crisis or war. In times other than congressional or presidential call-up, the National Guard falls under the governor of the state to which it is assigned with the adjutant general acting as the commander. Neither active nor reserve component service members may serve within the National Guard. National Guard duties are under the auspices of the U.S. Code, Title 32, working in state-level jobs.

Operation Iraqi Freedom had representation from all military components. One hundred seventy-five thousand (175,000) men and women from all five of the active U.S. Armed Forces (as well as the Coast Guard) and the seven armed forces reserves (Army Reserve, Army National Guard, Navy Reserve, Air Force Reserve, Air National Guard, Marine Corps Reserve, and Coast Guard Reserve) initially crossed into Iraq. In November 2003, the Vice Chief of Staff of the Army, General John M. Keane, identified a total force of 192,800 involved in Operation Iraqi Freedom: 133,000 Army, 550 Air Force, 1,550 Navy, 8,600 Marine, 12,400 Coalition, 2,400 Army Special Operations, and 34,000 Army forces in Kuwait.

With the recent decreasing size of the U.S. Armed Forces and increased numbers of assigned missions (both war and operations other than war), the tempo of operations (OPTEMPO) for active and reserve members has increased in frequency and intensity. It is expected that more military members will deploy to unaccompanied overseas assignments repeatedly during their careers. As such, many of those deployed in the current conflict may have been previously deployed and will likely deploy again.

ARMY

As the oldest branch of the U.S. Military, founded in 1775, the **Army** is one of the most powerful fighting forces on earth. Approximately 522,388 full-time soldiers in today's Army defend and serve our nation by land, sea, and air. Elite groups within the Army, such as the Army Rangers and Special Forces, receive specialized training for advanced combat situations. Today's **Army Reserve** is 189,000 troops strong and the **National Guard** consists of approximately 325,000 troops from all U.S. states and territories.

MARINE CORPS

The United States **Marine Corps** was founded in 1775, even before our nation was officially formed. While the Marine Corps is the smallest branch of today's military, it plays a major role as the first force on the ground in most conflicts. Today, over 200,000 marines are stationed around the world at all times, ready to deploy quickly whenever and wherever needed. The **Marine Corps Reserve** differs from other reserve branches in that it is made up primarily of marines formerly on active duty. There is practically no such thing as being a "retired" marine—the commitment is 24/7, and for life.

NAVY

The U.S. **Navy** was founded under the authority of George Washington in 1775, with the intent to intercept British supply ships near Massachusetts. Currently comprising 337,690 personnel, today's Navy is equipped to handle operations both on and under the sea, in the air, and on the ground. Its reach is worldwide, spanning one hundred international ports and touching the farthest corners of the open ocean. The **Navy Reserve** comprises more than 30 percent of total Navy assets and, when called to action, can be found abroad, on shore, in the air, or at sea. The Navy Reserve's involvement with the Navy continues to grow. Currently, 126,794 Navy Reservists stand by to join the fleet when needed as active parts of the largest and most powerful naval force in the world.

AIR FORCE

The **Air Force** began as a subdivision of the U.S. Army and was declared an official combatant arm in 1920. It wasn't until 1947, following World War II, that the Air Force was recognized as its own military branch.

Today's Air Force operates in keeping with a three-part vision: global vigilance, reach, and power. This vision empowers a technologically advanced force of 352,000 troops focused on air, space, and cyberspace superiority. The **Air Force Reserve** currently employs 74,000 trained reservists. Though this makes up 15 percent of the Air Force's overall manpower, the extent of their contribution is much greater. More than 30 percent of all Air Force missions are accomplished through the efforts of Air Force reservists. The **Air Guard** is an essential component of the U.S. Air Force. Currently, this force is made up of 160,700 Air Guard personnel. There are more than 140 Air Guard units throughout the United States and its territories.

COAST GUARD

The **Coast Guard** is an amalgamation of formerly distinct federal services: the U.S. Lighthouse Service, the Revenue Cutter Service, the Steamboat Inspection Service, and the U.S. Lifesaving Service. Today, the Coast Guard operates under the Department of Homeland Security during peacetime and under the Navy during wartime, or by special presidential order. In addition to protecting our nation's waterways, the 39,000 active-duty members of the Coast Guard perform search and rescue, law enforcement, and environmental cleanup operations. The **Coast Guard Reserve** has 8,100 reservists supporting and aiding critical Coast Guard missions.

CURRENT STATUS

ACTIVE DUTY

1.4 million service members are on active duty.

1.2 million service members are in the National Guard and the Military Reserve.

500,000 service members are stationed or deployed overseas.

VETERANS

24.4 million veterans.

2 million veterans are under age thirty-five.

1.7 million veterans are women.

1 in 4 adult males is a veteran.

Types of Conflict and Associated Stresses

During missions there are multiple stages and types of conflict. Throughout an operation, these stages can overlap depending on the location and mission of assigned forces. Each form of conflict may contribute to different forms or expressions of stress. It is therefore valuable to determine precisely the nature and duration of exposures for returning troops.

PRE-DEPLOYMENT PHASE

During the pre-deployment phase military members face uncertainty and worry. Deployment orders change routinely, sometimes with multiple revisions of deadlines and locations. Service members worry about the safety of themselves as well as their family members.

They struggle to ensure that finances, health care, child care, and pets all will be managed in their absence. In the current climate, deploying service members may have additional concerns about terrorist activities in the United States during the period of deployment. Pre-deployment can be extremely stressful on single parents, reserve forces, and military members who have not previously deployed. It is often difficult during this phase to determine the difference between reasonable anxiety and an excessive reaction or the development or recurrence of psychiatric illness.

DEPLOYMENT PHASE

The deployment phase carries many additional pressures. The stress of traditional, high-intensity warfare leads to fear and uncertainty. Operational plans change constantly; knowledge of enemy capabilities is unclear; equipment breaks down; and logistical supply lines are uncertain. Combatants face the threat of their own death or injury and also witness the death, wounding, and disfigurement of their companions, enemy forces, and civilians.

During this heightened physiologic state, the high level of emotion, and the intensity of sensory exposure may lead to heightened levels of arousal, attempts to avoid emotion, and intrusive recollections of events. The novelty of the situation may also contribute to symptoms of dissociation. The severity and duration of symptoms will vary among individuals. This phase of combat is highly conducive to acute stress disorder and post-traumatic stress disorder in military members.

TYPES OF CONFLICT

Low-intensity combat is typical during peacemaking and peacekeeping missions. Fear of death or injury is less imminent, but chronically present. Some troops may intermittently encounter the exposures found in high-intensity combat. The majority will experience chronic strain of deployment: family separation, heat, cold, harsh living conditions, extremely long duty hours with little respite, minimal communication with the outside world, and boredom. These strains can result in the development of adjustment disorders, mood disorders, anxiety disorders, and exacerbations of personality disorders. Some members with predisposing factors may develop psychotic disorders. Depending on the availability of substances of abuse, abuse or dependence disorders may develop, recur, or worsen (Jones, 1995a).

Terrorist activities and guerilla warfare tactics, such as car bombings, remotely detonated explosives, and mortar attacks lead to chronic strain and anxiety. Psychologically this can contribute to service members questioning their purpose, as well as negative attributions about the importance and need for the sacrifices encountered. Coupled with other exposures, exposure during this phase may exacerbate illness or delay recovery. Many of the veterans from prior wars have focused on their discontent associated with sacrifice and loss in a mission viewed as unpopular and unsuccessful.

In a highly armed nation such as Iraq or Afghanistan, U.S. troops cannot be certain whether an innocent-appearing civilian may be carrying a firearm, an explosive, or a remote detonation device. Rules of engagement are altered regularly by command in response to political and tactical requirements.

When an individual or a vehicle challenges a roadblock or security checkpoint, a delay in the use of force may result in friendly forces injuries. A premature response may result in the unnecessary death of civilians. Such conditions create chronic strain, particularly when split-second decisions may undergo retrospective analyses to determine their appropriateness (Jones, 1995b).

Friendly fire events are among the most tragic. In the current military environment of high-technology communication, command, and control, there is a much lower risk of such occurrences. When they take place it is usually when there are failures of communication between allied forces. To date, no major events have occurred during Operation Iraqi Freedom, but they have occurred during Operation Enduring Freedom, the war in Afghanistan. Similar to terrorist and guerilla acts, friendly fire incidents (either by those responsible for or those who experienced the act) also lead to negative attributions about purpose of mission and specifically about the failure of leadership in preventing such outcomes. Friendly fire incidents can be more difficult for service members to cognitively reconstruct, leading to less opportunity for integration and potentially greater traumatic impact.

Clinical assessment must not assume that the experiences of all service members coming out of Iraq or Afghanistan are identical. Exposure to military conflict can be of a variety of types and intensities. A careful assessment should ensure that there is a complete understanding of all pre-deployment and deployment happenings. As a military patient may be reluctant to share details of his or her experiences early on with an unfamiliar provider, a thoughtful and detailed accounting of experiences will likely require the time to develop a trusting therapeutic relationship. As is clear from the information presented above, a service member's emotional response to wartime exposures is determined by specific experiences, but equally important is the context in which these experiences are encountered and the meanings they hold.

MILITARY MEDICAL EVACUATION AND SERVICE DELIVERY

It is important to understand the echelons of medical care and evacuation when treating the combat veteran to understand the early interventions available and the limitations of far-forward treatments. Medical care is provided through the continuum of up to five echelons of care.

The Combat Stress Control doctrine promotes the PIES principle in the management of battle fatigue casualties: Proximity of treatment close to the front, Immediacy of treatment, Expectancy of return to duty (RTD), and

Simplicity of intervention. Those who do not respond to early interventions are evacuated to the next echelon based on the capabilities and evacuation policy established by the command surgeon.

Echelons of Care

Echelon I care is the treatment provided by the medical assets organic to the combat unit. Veterans who experience combat trauma will likely be attended by members of their own battalion. A veteran who has sustained a physical battle injury will receive first aid by his or her buddy and the unit medic. Initial care will focus on maintaining an airway, controlling bleeding, and preventing shock with intravenous fluids and field dressing. The veteran will be transported by air or ground ambulance to the Battalion Aid Station to be stabilized for further evacuation.

Echelon II care is provided at the brigade and division level. Emergency medical treatment, including resuscitation, is continued and the patient is stabilized for further transport. This level includes the farthest forward Combat Stress Control (CSC) elements available to address combat stress issues. Resources in the Division Support Area include the Division Mental Health Section (DMHS), consisting of a psychiatrist, psychologist, social worker, and enlisted behavioral science specialists; and a CSC detachment with additional providers, nurses, and enlisted staff. The DMHS role is to provide command-consultation, preventive services, treatment, and screening while the CSC augments treatment and screening and provides a holding capacity for respite and reconstitution. Brief supportive therapy and pharmacologic intervention are doctrinally available at this level. In practice, these treatments are variably present depending upon geographic, personnel, and logistical limitations.

Echelon III care is provided at the forward deployed Combat Support Hospitals (CSHs) located in the Corps Support Area. These hospitals are staffed and equipped to provide resuscitation, initial wound surgery, and postoperative treatment. Inpatient and outpatient psychiatric care is available in the CSH, but the extent of available medical and psychiatric staffing may vary depending upon the organization of each CSH. As this is the first echelon of care where a fully staffed pharmacy exists, antipsychotic, anxiolytic, and antidepressant medications are usually obtainable. Patients are treated at this level to the extent they can be managed within the guidelines of the theater aeromedical evacuation policy. Recent policy in Iraq has been that patients who are not expected to respond to treatment and return to duty within seven days are to be evacuated out of theater. Psychiatrists at the CSHs in Iraq and Kuwait report that more than 90 percent of service members are treated and returned to duty.

Echelon IV consists of hospitals staffed and equipped for general and specialized medical and surgical care as well as reconditioning and rehabilitation for return to duty (RTD). These facilities are generally located outside the combat zone. Iraq veterans are evacuated to Landstuhl Regional Medical Center in Germany or U.S. Naval Hospital, Rota, Spain. Service members evacuated to this echelon are rarely returned to duty.

Echelon V is the definitive medical care provided in continental U.S. Military and Veterans Affairs Medical Centers. Experience shows that the RTD rate for troops evacuated to the continental United States (CONUS) with disorders ranging from adjustment disorders, depression, anxiety, acute stress disorder (ASD), and post-traumatic stress disorder (PTSD) is extremely low. Aggressive treatment of symptoms seeks to induce remission with the goal of retaining the military member in the military through stabilization at the unit's rear detachment, a demobilization station, or the medical center. Military patients whose symptoms cannot be resolved must be considered for referral to a Medical Evaluation Board (discussed later in this book).

MEDICAL EVACUATION

At each echelon, the veteran is evaluated for ability to RTD. The mobility of units on the modern battlefield and the need for service members to be able to sustain the extraordinary demands of high OPTEMPO diminish the likelihood of returning someone to his or her unit. Commanders require military members to perform at full capacity; as such they are frequently reticent to reintegrate a combat stress casualty to the unit. This preference often is balanced by a commander's need to maintain sufficient manpower for combat readiness. As insomnia is the most common initial complaint of a military member referred to mental health providers, commanders will often allow a time-limited medication trial to determine if the individual will rapidly respond and be available for missions. Contemporary battlefield realities, however, create an environment in which the validity and feasibility of the PIES concept must be seriously rethought.

Reports from psychiatrists deployed to Iraq suggest that when a psychiatrically distressed service member is able to stay with his or her unit and is afforded modified duty for a limited time, PIES remains effective. With each level of evacuation, the military patient becomes more removed from the unit. Experience demonstrates that once evacuated from the CSH a soldier is unlikely to be returned to combat. Combat stress casualties often begin to experience relief of some acute symptoms when removed from the combat trauma. This relief is a potent reinforcer, serving to make the soldier apprehensive about his or her ability to tolerate reexposure. This confluence of factors creates powerful forces in the direction of evacuation and diminishes the likelihood of returning the military member to combat duty.

Military patients processed through the evacuation system will have various modalities of treatment, ranging from supportive measures to fairly intensive treatment. It will vary in accordance with the patient, the diagnosis, disposition, and the availability of treatment at the various locations. By the time the patient has arrived in CONUS he or she will have had several screens and some level of specialized care throughout the evacuation and disposition process.

PSYCHIATRIC DISORDERS SEEN DURING WARTIME

The destructive force of war creates an atmosphere of chaos and compels service members to face the terror of unexpected injury, loss, and death. The combat environment (austere living conditions, heavy physical demands, sleep deprivation, periods of intense violence followed by unpredictable periods of relative inactivity, separation from loved ones, etc.) is itself a psychological stressor that may precipitate a wide range of emotional distress and/ or psychiatric disorders. Psychological injury may occur as a consequence of physical injury, disruption of the environment, fear, rage, or helplessness produced by combat, or a combination of these factors.

The psychiatric differential diagnosis for military patients at war is quite broad. The clinical picture will vary over the course of a war depending on individual characteristics (e.g., personality traits, coping skills, and prior illness), available social supports, and the amount of time that has passed between clinical presentation and the precipitating event(s). Thus, it is useful to consider the range of emotional responses in the context of the multiphasic traumatic stress response:

- Immediate phase characterized by strong emotions, disbelief, numbness, fear, and confusion accompanied by symptoms of autonomic arousal and anxiety
- Delayed phase characterized by persistence of autonomic arousal, intrusive recollections, somatic symptoms, and combinations of anger, mourning, apathy, and social withdrawal
- Chronic phase including continued intrusive symptoms and arousal for some, disappointment or resentment or sadness for others, and for the majority a refocus on new challenges and the rebuilding of lives (Benedek et al., 2001; Ursano et al., 1994)

Within this three-phase framework of traumatic response, symptoms noted in the immediate phase of combat generally reflect either predictable "normal" individual response to extreme stressors (e.g., psychic distress not meeting threshold criteria for DSM-IV-TR [*Diagnostic and Statistical Manual of Mental Disorders*, fourth edition, text revision] psychiatric disorders— "battle fatigue" or "combat stress" in military parlance), exacerbations of preexisting conditions, or neuropsychiatric effects insults. These insults might include exposure to trauma, the central nervous system (CNS) effects (e.g., delirium) of chemical, biological (Franz et al., 1997; DiGiovanni, 1999), or other naturally occurring infectious agents, head or internal injury from missiles, blast effects, or other projectiles. ASD or adjustment disorders may manifest themselves in the immediacy of combat and, as with other forms of trauma or disaster, exacerbations of substance abuse, depression, or preexisting PTSD (Schlenger et al., 2002; Shuster et al., 2001; Vlahov et al., 2002) may also occur. As personality disorders are, by definition, pervasive patterns of maladaptive response to stress, the stress of war can certainly precipitate exacerbations of previously subclinical personality disorders or maladaptive traits.

In the delayed phase following intense operational stressors, PTSD, substance abuse, and somatization disorder (or multiple unexplained physical symptoms) may be observed, and persistent anger, irritability, or sadness may signal major depressive disorder or other mood disorders. Symptoms of bereavement or traumatic grief may also occur as service members reflect on the loss of brothers-in-arms. Troops provide significant support to one another during war, so such losses may have as much emotional impact as the loss of a close relative and may be accompanied by feelings of guilt—particularly if the lost service member was a "battle buddy."

While a "fight or flight" instinct may preempt self-injurious behavior during the height of battle, anxiety symptoms, social withdrawal, and depressed mood may occur during the delayed phase and increase the risk for self-injury or suicide during this phase. To the extent that the military member received psychological support from comrades before and during battle, medical evacuation (due to physical injury or neuropsychiatric symptoms) may disrupt the support of the service member, compounding the risk of self-injury.

During the chronic phase some service members will experience persistent PTSD symptoms or the more subtle secondary effect of exposure to chemical or biological agents (or their antidotes). These secondary effects include depression, personality changes, or cognitive dysfunction (DiGiovanni, 1999). Dysthymic disorder, mixed subsyndromal depression/anxiety or subclinical PTSD may evolve and substance use disorders may become more firmly entrenched. For some military patients with PTSD, the pervasive distrust, irritability, and sense of foreshortened future may have more debilitating effects on social and occupational function than intrusive symptoms. Indeed the avoidance of reminders of the trauma (a symptom of PTSD) may result in affected individuals declining exposure-based therapy, or any treatment whatsoever, thus compounding not only the impact of war-related pathology but any preexistent illness as well.

In summary, no single psychiatric diagnosis characterizes the service member's response to war. For many, the training, comradery, unity of purpose, individual coping skills, and mutual support provided by comrades may protect against the development of severe psychiatric disorders as a consequence of war. However, even individuals who do not develop symptoms meeting criteria for DSM-IV disorders may react with transient changes in mood, affect, cognition, or combinations of these and somatic symptoms typically termed "battle fatigue." They may require psychological support at one point or intermittently during a campaign as a result of their individual response to particular events or their operational environment. For others, ASD or the neuropsychiatric sequelae of head trauma or exposure to toxic agents may occur. Major depressive disorder and other affective disorders, bereavement, substance abuse disorders, and somatoform disorders may also occur over time (see table 1.1). Although PTSD may not be the most com-

Table 1.1

Phase	Description	Diagnostic Considerations
Immediate	During or immediately after traumatic event(s): strong emotions, disbelief, numbness, fear, confusion, anxiety, autonomic arousal	Battle fatigue, delirium (from toxic exposures, head injury), acute stress disorder, adjustment disorders, brief psychotic disorder, exacerbation of substance abuse, personality disorders or traits, or premorbid mood, anxiety, or thought disorders
Delayed	Approximately one week after trauma or in the aftermath of combat: intrusive thoughts, autonomic arousal (startle, insomnia, nightmares, irritability), somatic symptoms, grief/mourning, apathy, social withdrawal	PTSD, substance abuse, somatoform disorders, depression, other mood and anxiety disorders, bereavement
Chronic	Months to years after: disappointment or resentment, sadness, persistent intrusive symptoms, refocus on new life events	PTSD, chronic effects of toxic exposure, dysthymic disorder, other mood disorders, substance abuse disorders, emotional recovery—perspective

mon emotional response to war, symptoms such as dissociation and avoidance of reminders of trauma (which may be adaptive, or may occur as associated features of other war-related illnesses) may impede treatment efforts of PTSD or other syndromes. Given the wide range of potential disorders or symptoms of distress that may evolve over time, the difficulty in distinguishing acute adaptive responses from psychopathology, and our inability to predict who may be most severely affected over time, initial interventions should be aimed at ensuring safety to self and others and developing mechanisms to monitor symptoms over time and encourage access to care.

2

Blast Injuries and Concussions

BLAST INJURIES

America's armed forces are sustaining attacks from explosions or blast by rocket-propelled grenades, improvised explosive devices (IEDs), and land mines almost daily in deployed settings. Civilian workers and military personnel working in these combat zones are at increased risk of blast-related trauma, particularly blast-related traumatic brain injury (TBI).

Some of the TBI and concussive injuries associated with significant blast may not be identified accurately for several reasons. Initially, the blast-related TBI or concussion may have occurred simultaneously with other more obvious life-threatening injuries. Initially, the focus of medical care providers must be on the most life-threatening injuries. Sometimes, in the case of a concussion/mild TBI (mTBI) resulting from blast, there may be no outward sign of injury; service members may also be reluctant to endorse acute symptoms because they do not want to be medically evacuated and separated from their unit. Because blast exposure is so common in the combat zones and almost everyone has had some of the acute symptoms of concussion, it may not be identified as problematic until the service member returns home from the deployment.

Finally, concussions and TBI related to significant blast exposure are also likely to have other important comorbid conditions present. For example, the patient may also have combat stress or depression associated with a return from deployment; it is very challenging for the medical providers in these situations to determine which symptoms are due to the concussion and which symptoms are due to the combat stress or depression.

How Does Blast Exposure Cause a Concussion or a
Traumatic Brain Injury?

A TBI is caused by a blow or jolt to the head or a penetrating head injury that disrupts the function of the brain. Exposure to blast events can affect the body in a number of ways; in addition, these different injuries mechanisms can interact and result in more impairments or prolonged periods of recovery.

- Primary blast injury is the result of exposure to the overpressurization wave or the complex pressure wave that is generated by the blast itself. This blast overpressurization wave travels at a high velocity and is affected by the surrounding environment; for example, the effects of the blast wave may be increased in a closed environment such as a vehicle. Air-filled organs such as the ear, lung, and gastrointestinal tract and organs surrounded by fluid-filled cavities such as the brain and spinal cord are especially susceptible to primary blast injury (Elsayed, 1997; Mayorga, 1997). The overpressurization wave dissipates quickly, causing the greatest risk of injury to those closest to the explosion.
- Secondary blast injury is the result of energized fragments flying through the air; these fragments may cause penetrating brain injury.
- Tertiary blast injury may occur when the individual is thrown from the blast into a solid object such as an adjacent wall or even a steering wheel. These types of injuries are associated with acceleration/deceleration forces and blunt force trauma to the brain similar to that observed following high speed motor vehicle accidents.
- Finally, quaternary blast injury can occur in the presence of severe blast-related trauma resulting from significant blood loss associated with traumatic amputations or even from inhalation of toxic gases resulting from the explosion.

TBI resulting from blast exposure can be much more complex compared to TBI from other causes. As such, it is challenging to differentiate blast-related TBI and/or concussion from other conditions. Finally, it is also difficult to estimate the course of recovery in these cases, as it may vary widely depending on various types of blast injury and other injury variables, such as the size of the blast, distance from the blast, and so on. Because of these issues, it may be difficult to assess blast-related TBI and concussion in the same manner that other brain injuries are examined. A better approach may be to conduct an evaluation based on the mechanism (cause) of the injury; that is, screen all individual service members exposed to a blast for any symptoms that might be resulting from the effects of blast on the brain.

What Symptoms May Indicate a Blast-Related Brain Injury?

Difficulties experienced as a result of a closed brain blast injury may include a range of physical, emotional, cognitive, and behavioral symptoms. Many of these symptoms are nonspecific however; that is, they occur with other conditions such as depression or combat stress. It requires an experience clinician who is familiar with the many variables involved in blast injury and has an understanding of how these variables can affect recovery and ultimately impact return to everyday activities.

What Is DVBIC Doing to Care for Those with Blast Injuries?

The Defense and Veterans Brain Injury Center (DVBIC) works to identify all service members who have sustained a closed brain injury during combat operations and to ensure that they receive the best care available. Because the effects of blast injury on the brain are still being discovered, DVBIC has led the way in developing a number of important research projects examining specific variables involved in the blast. In addition, DVBIC has been involved in studies on developing combat gear which will better protect the brain should a blast occur.

Finally, DVBIC has been involved in the validation of several important diagnostic tests for better identifying the blast effects on the brain; these include the use of advanced neuroimaging techniques, such as diffuse tensor-weighted imaging (DTI) and advanced technologies for measuring the function of the brain as the individual works on specific tasks; this technique is known as magnetoencephalography (MEG).

BLAST INJURY BASICS: A PRIMER FOR THE MEDICAL SPEECH-LANGUAGE PATHOLOGIST

Gloriajean L. Wallace, *The ASHA Leader*[1]

Each era is associated with a unique pattern of wartime injuries. In this century, a new and highly sophisticated pattern of missile warfare exposes service members and civilian survivors of terrorist attacks to explosions which cause strong air-pressure "blasts." Multi-level injury from blast exposure, referred to as "blast injury," may result in a constellation of impairments to body organs and systems. The multiorgan/multisystem involvement, known as "polytrauma," adds significant complexity to the medical and rehabilitation profile for individuals who survive blast injury.

Medical speech-language pathologists (SLPs) are well-prepared to provide services to patients with traumatic brain injury (TBI); aphasia; motor speech impairment; dysphagia; oral, facial, oral-pharyngeal, nasal-pharyngeal, and laryngeal trauma; and hearing loss. However, medical SLPs are now faced with providing services to an increasing number of patients who simultaneously may have some or all of these conditions.

As a result, medical SLPs face challenges in treating this population, particularly in the area of clinical management considerations such as prioritization and sequencing of treatment focus and the impact of impairments in one treatment area on rehabilitation efforts in another. To promote seamless continuity of care from military to community settings for these individuals and quality care for civilian survivors, it will be necessary for medical SLPs to prepare themselves to provide clinical services and to serve as community reentry advocates for survivors of blast injury.

An understanding of blast injury basics provides clarity regarding the risk for polytrauma and the resulting communication and swallowing impairments that may be encountered by medical SLPs providing services to this population.

Effects of Blast Exposure

The term "blast injury" refers to injury from barotraumas caused by either an over-pressurization or under-pressurization of air over normal atmospheric pressure that affects the body's surface due to exposure to detonated devices or weapons. A phenomenon called "blast overpressure" forms from the compression of air in front of a blast wave, which heats and accelerates the movement of air molecules. This overpressure phenomenon is considered to be the positive phase of the blast wave.

The negative phase of the blast wave occurs later, as a result of sub-atmospheric pressure/underpressurization. The amount of damage from the pressure wave depends on the peak pressure, duration, medium in which the explosion occurs (open air, confined space, or water), and distance from the explosion. Air- and fluid-filled organs are especially susceptible to the over-pressurization/underpressurization effects of blast waves—which cause the primary effects of blast exposure. Pulmonary barotraumas, tympanic membrane rupture and middle ear damage, abdominal hemorrhage, perforation of the globe of the eye, and concussion (TBI without physical sign of head injury) are some of the primary effects of blast exposure.

The secondary effects of blast injury result from flying debris such as bomb fragments, and can result in eye penetration, open head brain injury, and a variety of other medical problems. The tertiary effects of blast injury result from the individual being thrown by the blast wind, and can cause fracture, traumatic amputation, closed and open brain injury, and a host of other medical problems. The quaternary (or miscellaneous) effects of blast injury refer to all explosion-related injuries, illnesses, or diseases not due to primary, secondary or tertiary mechanisms. These includes burns, crush injuries, closed and open head brain injury, angina, hyperglycemia, hypertension, and asthma and other breathing problems resulting from the inhalation of dust, smoke, or toxic fumes.

Explosives

The type of explosive will have an impact on the nature and severity of the resulting blast injury. Explosives are categorized as either "high-order" or "low-order." High-order explosives are chemicals which have a high rate of reaction—including nitroglycerin, dynamite, C-4, and a mixture of ammonium nitrate and fuel oil. When a high-order explosive detonates, the chemicals are converted into gas at a very high temperature and pressure. High-order explosives have the potential to generate a large volume of initial pressure, and a blast wave that may expand outwards in all directions.

Low-order explosives are designed to burn and gradually release energy at a relatively slow rate. This type of explosive (including pipe bombs, gunpowder, and "Molotov cocktails") are referred to as "propellants" because they propel an object such as a bullet through a barrel. Low-order explosives do not create the shock waves generated by high-order explosives. The "blast wind" of low-order explosives is a "pushing" rather than the "shattering" effect found in the "blast wave" of high-order explosives. Injuries resulting from low-order explosives are typically caused by fragments of the container, blast wind from expanding gases, and thermal injuries associated with the heat of the explosion.

Additional factors that affect the nature and severity of blast-related injuries include the container in which the explosive is housed, the barriers between the explosive and the person, the distance from the explosion, and the space around the explosion (whether it occurred in an enclosed or an open space). Protective gear such as Kevlar also affects injury severity. It includes a helmet, neck gear, and protective vest that shields the abdomen and groin area.

A Long Road

Communication disorders resulting from blast injury can include cognitive communication impairments related to TBI, swallowing impairments, aphasia, motor speech impairment, oral and facial burns or other trauma, smoke inhalation and resulting laryngeal trauma, medical conditions requiring trach and vent, and hearing loss. Although the patient is at risk for communication disorders in all these areas, TBI poses the greatest risk because it may be caused by all four mechanisms (primary, secondary, tertiary and quandary) of blast injury.

Patients with combat-related injuries receive initial immediate care by "Forward Surgical Teams" who remain directly behind the troops in preparedness for the provision of needed medical attention. The injured are then sent to the Combat Support Hospital and then are evacuated to a Level IV Hospital in one of the following locations: Kuwait; Rota, Spain (Naval Hospital); or Landstuhl, Germany (Army Hospital).

If medical care requiring more than thirty days is needed, the injured are transferred to a U.S. military hospital—Walter Reed Army Medical Center, National Naval Medical Center (WRAMC), or Brooke Army Medical Center, which specializes in burn treatment. Those who will not return to combat and still require rehabilitation will next be seen at a VA Hospital and ultimately a civilian/community-based facility.

Patients who survive blast injury may incur traditional open head brain injury (secondary effects), closed head brain injury (tertiary effects), and brain injury from the primary "blast overpressurization" phenomenon (cerebral contusion). Indirect brain injury due to resulting air embolism (and stroke) may also result from blast overpressurization (incidence unknown). Blast overpressurization exposure adds significant complexity to the profile of blast cases with TBI, which may prove to be an important research area.

Because of exposure to traumatic events, the loss of health and independence, and bodily disfigurement that blast cases may encounter, these cases are at risk for a host of psychiatric disorders, including post-traumatic stress disorder (PTSD). Many PTSD symptoms overlap with symptoms of TBI, especially mild brain injury: headache, dizziness, irritability, decreased concentration, memory problems, fatigue, visual disturbances, sensitivity to light and noise, judgment problems, anxiety, and depression. Similarities in the behavioral characteristics of patients with TBI and/or PTSD can complicate the rehabilitation team's diagnostic assessment effort.

The road to recovery for individuals who have incurred blast injuries is a long and complicated one. Medical SLPs must prepare to provide clinical services and to serve as community re-entry advocates for survivors of blast injury.

Successful community reintegration will require the intervention of medical and rehabilitation professionals who are knowledgeable, committed, and caring. I challenge you to explore this emerging area further to determine the role that you can play in facilitating restoration and wholeness to returning warriors and others who have survived the ravages of blast injury.

*   *   *

CONCUSSIONS

Sports Concussion and Combat Blast Injury

Jeffrey T. Barth, Ph.D.

Up until the early 1980s it was believed that most mild head injured patients made rapid and complete recoveries. Then evidence began to accumulate supporting the notion that these injuries could be problematic for a minority of patients. Return to work was delayed, and symptoms such as fatigue, headaches, depression, irritability, cognitive slowing, and problems with attention, learning, and memory were noted in a small percentage of mild head injured patients three months post injury. These persistent symptoms were part of the post-concussion syndrome (PCS) constellation.

In the mid-1980s, in a unique attempt to control for individual variability and understand mild head injury in civilian populations (motor vehicle accidents, falls, etc.), the University of Virginia began using Sports as a Laboratory Assessment Model (SLAM) to study concussion and what was being termed mild traumatic brain injury (mTBI)/concussion. These investigations of college football players, which involved brief baseline and repeat post-concussion neurocognitive assessments, revealed that blunt trauma and/or acceleration-deceleration injury to the head, with alteration of consciousness (yet no true loss of consciousness) can result in neurocognitive deficits in attention, concentration, learning, memory, and processing speed, as well as symptoms such as headache and dizziness. They found that with rest, young, healthy, bright, motivated athletes recover within five to ten days of injury, and sometimes much more rapidly, after a single concussion. Since these original studies, other investigators have noted similar findings across contact sports.

Multiple concussions pose a more complex problem. There is a growing literature and case examples of more severe trauma associated with multiple concussions in sports, as well as a lowering of the threshold for incurring additional concussions. Although rare, returning to play before complete recovery from concussion and sustaining a second concussion can result in a catastrophic neurological injury referred to as second-impact syndrome (SIS).

An unexpected benefit of this sports concussion research was that it provided the first empirical data for the development of return to play (RTP) guidelines and decision-making for reducing poor outcome. For example, when using the American Academy of Neurology (AAN) severity and RTP guidelines, if a player were to sustain his or her first mild (grade I) concussion and all symptoms were to subside (with physical exertion) within fifteen minutes, they might be allowed to return to play that day. If the symptoms lasted more than fifteen minutes (grade II concussion), the player would be held out of play and practice for one week post-symptom resolution.

In the war in Iraq and Afghanistan, improvised explosive devices create blast injuries, which are the most common cause of TBI in the theater of combat. Mild and moderate TBIs are more prevalent in this conflict due to the vast improvement in protective gear worn by our service members. Blast injuries can result in the full spectrum of closed and penetrating TBIs (mild, moderate, and severe). The mild to moderate blast-related TBIs are often overlooked in the presence of more severe polytrauma. Blast injuries are defined by four potential mechanism dynamics:

1. Primary Blast: Atmospheric overpressure followed by underpressure or vacuum.
2. Secondary Blast: Objects placed in motion by the blast hitting the service member.
3. Tertiary Blast: Service member being placed in motion by the blast.

4. Quaternary Blast: Other injuries from the blast such as burns, crush injuries, toxic fumes.

The Defense and Veterans Brain Injury Center (DVBIC), in its efforts to assess and manage these blast injuries in theater and at all other levels of care, brought military and civilian head injury and sports medicine experts together to facilitate a dialog on mTBI /concussion, since there are clear similarities between these sports concussions and combat blast injuries. The similarities lie in the secondary and tertiary blast dynamics of blunt trauma and acceleration-deceleration injury.

The physical and neurocognitive symptoms associated with these blast injuries are also very similar to the sequelae of sports concussions and mTBI in motor vehicle accidents. Blast injury, however, is more complex than sports concussion, given the overpressure and underpressure atmospheric dynamics and the quaternary collateral trauma.

Nevertheless, DVBIC and its civilian partners recognized the usefulness of using a variation on the sports concussion model for use in theater with these blast injuries, and they developed Clinical Practice Guidelines for the Assessment and Management of Concussion and mTBI. These guidelines offer brief screening techniques (MACE: Military Acute Concussion Evaluation) adapted from those used to identify sports concussion on the athletic field (SAC: Standardized Assessment of Concussion). They also proposed consensus driven return to duty (RTD) guidelines, which were again similar to the RTP sports guidelines (rest and return when symptom free).

Although blast injury dynamics is more complex and often more severe than sports concussion, and it appears that multiple blast traumas are much more common than multiple sports concussions, the lessons learned from sports medicine have paved the way for a better understanding of combat TBI. There is a new awareness of the potential concussion problem associated with blast injury, brief baseline neurocognitive assessments have been initiated predeployment for many of our troops, and guidelines are in place to help all health care providers, from the medic to the surgeon, in the appropriate assessment and management of this combat injury.

Cumulative Concussions

Cumulative or repetitive concussion is most widely studied in the world of sports medicine. Researchers investigating the relationship between blast exposure and concussion are currently looking to see if findings from sports medicine can be translated to the military population.

A National Collegiate Athletic Association (NCAA) football study (Guskiewicz et al. 2003) found an association between the number of reported prior concussions in NCAA football players and the likelihood of sustaining another concussion. The study found that players reporting more than three prior concussions were 3 times more likely to sustain another concussion than players who reported no prior concussions. Among players reporting two prior concussions they were 2.5 times more likely to sustain another concussion. Players that reported only one prior concussion were 1.4 times more likely to sustain another concussion. The study also found that a prior history of concussion may be associated with slower recovery of neurological function. After a concussion, players most commonly complained of headache, dizziness/balance difficulties, and feeling cognitively "slowed down." Players who have sustained prior concussions should be educated regarding their increased risk of repeat concussions when continuing to play contact sports. This same study also suggested that a history of concussion is associated with prolonged recovery following future concussions.

A worst-case scenario is a rare complication called "second-impact syndrome" caused by sustaining a second concussion before the symptoms of the prior concussion have resolved. This condition can be fatal.

There is conflicting data regarding the cumulative pathologic effects of multiple concussions. There is also no consensus on how many concussions are too many, in either the sports world or the military.

NOTE

1. Gloriajean Wallace is a medical speech-language pathologist and professor in the Department of Communication Sciences and Disorders at the University of Cincinnati.

3

Traumatic Brain Injury

One of the most difficult things about having a TBI is that people do not always have immediate symptoms. Also, sometimes the symptoms are present but not obvious. TBIs are common wounds in OEF/OIF because of the frequent exposure to improvised explosive device (IED) blasts. The protective gear issued now is better than in previous wars. For instance, many who were exposed to blasts in Vietnam and in previous conflicts or wars did not survive.

The percentage of brain injury in Vietnam was 14 to 18 percent. Today, the survival rate is higher, but so is the brain-injury level. The newer complication is that while the body is protected, especially with the Kevlar helmets, the brain is literally shaken inside the protective brain sac. Blast injuries create extreme differences in air pressure, typically a thousand times greater than normal pressure, with a travel velocity of 1,600 feet per second. These shock waves that travel through the brain create small bubbles. Eventually these bubbles pop, leaving pockets or holes in the brain, similar to the holes found in baby Swiss cheese. Some authors have named this phenomenon "ghost shrapnel." If these bubbles occur inside blood vessels, they can form a blocked area, preventing oxygen from reaching that part of the brain, and killing that section of the brain. Shock waves can also cause bruising and hemorrhaging in certain areas of the brain, killing surrounding cells. The level of damage is impacted by where you are in relation to the path of the shock waves, how you are situated in that path, the rate of the rise of pressure, and the length of the pressure wave, or the time frame.

Current reports indicate that approximately 20 percent of OEF/OIF vets have been diagnosed with TBI, and 40 percent of those diagnosed cases have received care. Walter Reed Army Medical Center has reported that 31 percent of the people admitted there between early 2003 through mid-2005 had some level of TBI. It is thought that there are many more cases of service members with brain injuries that have yet to be diagnosed. While the percentages do not look greatly different from those from Vietnam, the level and type of brain injury is quite different. Many service members are deployed multiple times within theater, greatly increasing their chance of getting more than one concussion.

WHAT IS A TRAUMATIC BRAIN INJURY?

A traumatic brain injury (TBI) is a blow or jolt to the head or a penetrating head injury that disrupts the function of the brain. Not all blows or jolts to the head result in a TBI. The severity of such an injury may range from "mild"—a brief change in mental status or consciousness—to "severe," an extended period of unconsciousness or amnesia after the injury. A TBI can result in short- or long-term problems with independent function.

Traumatic brain injury is a significant health issue which affects service members and veterans during times of both peace and war. The high rate of TBI and blast-related concussion events resulting from current combat operations directly impacts the health and safety of individual service members and subsequently the level of unit readiness and troop retention. The impacts of TBI are felt within each branch of the service and throughout both the Department of Defense (DoD) and the Department of Veterans Affairs (VA) health care systems.

In the VA, TBI has become a major focus secondary to recognition of the need for increased resources to provide health care and vocational retraining for individuals with a diagnosis of TBI, as they transition to veteran status. Veterans may sustain TBIs throughout their lifespan, with the largest increase as the veterans enter into their seventies and eighties; these injuries are often due to falls and result in high levels of disability.

Active duty and reserve service members are at increased risk for sustaining a TBI compared to their civilian peers. This is a result of several factors, including the specific demographics of the military; in general, young men between the ages of eighteen and twenty-four are at greatest risk for TBI. Many operational and training activities which are routine in the military are physically demanding and even potentially dangerous. Military service members are increasingly deployed to areas where they are at risk for experiencing blast exposures from improvised explosive devices (IEDs), suicide bombers, land mines, mortar rounds, rocket-propelled grenades, and so on. These and other combat-related activities put our military service members at increased risk for sustaining a TBI.

Although recent attention has been intensively focused on combat-related TBI, it should be noted that TBI is not uncommon even in garrison and occurs during unusual daily activities; service members enjoy exciting leisure activities; they ride motorcycles, climb mountains, and parachute from planes for recreation. In addition, physical training is an integral part of the active duty service member's everyday life. These activities are expected for our service members and contribute to a positive quality of life, but these activities can also increase risk for TBI.

The following sections delve deeper into issues of TBI and the military. Topics aim to increase awareness of the unique issues which contribute to TBI in the military and what is being done to support the care and recovery of combat-wounded troops and veterans with TBI.

Traumatic brain injury (TBI) occurs from a sudden blow or jolt to the head. Brain injury often occurs during some type of trauma, such as an accident, blast, or a fall. Often when people refer to TBI, they are mistakenly talking about the symptoms that occur following a TBI. Actually, a TBI is the injury, not the symptoms.

What Causes TBI?

Not all blows or jolts to the head result in a TBI. The severity of such an injury may range from "mild"—a brief change in mental status or consciousness—to "severe," an extended period of unconsciousness or amnesia after the injury. The terms "concussion" and "mild TBI" (mTBI) are interchangeable.

In the military the leading causes of TBI are

- Bullets, fragments, blasts
- Falls
- Motor vehicle traffic crashes
- Assaults

Blasts are a leading cause of TBI for active duty military personnel in war zones.

Who Is at Highest Risk for TBI?

- Males are about 1.5 times as likely as females to sustain a TBI.
- Military duties increase the risk of sustaining a TBI.

How Serious Is My Injury?

A TBI is basically the same thing as a concussion. A TBI can be mild, moderate, or severe. These terms tell you the nature of the injury itself. They do not tell you what symptoms you may have or how severe the symptoms will be.

A TBI can occur even when there is no direct contact to the head. For example, when a person suffers whiplash, the brain may be shaken within the skull. This damage can cause bleeding between the brain and skull. Bruises can form where the brain hits the skull. Like bruises on other parts of the body, for mild injuries these will heal with time.

About 80 percent of all TBIs in civilians are mild (mTBI). Most people who have an mTBI will be back to normal by three months without any special treatment. Even patients with moderate or severe TBI can make remarkable recoveries.

The length of time that a person is unconscious (knocked out) is one way to measure how severe the injury was. If you weren't knocked out at all or if you were out for less than thirty minutes, your TBI was most likely minor or mild. If you were knocked out for more than thirty minutes but less than six hours, your TBI was most likely moderate.

What Are the Common Symptoms Following a TBI?

Symptoms that result from TBI are known as post-concussion syndrome (PCS). Few people will have all of the symptoms, but even one or two of the symptoms can be unpleasant. PCS makes it hard to work, get along at home, or relax. In the days, weeks, and months following a TBI the most common symptoms are

Physical
- Headache
- Feeling dizzy
- Being tired
- Trouble sleeping

- Vision problems
- Feeling bothered by noise and light

Cognitive (Mental)
- Memory problems
- Trouble staying focused
- Poor judgment and acting without thinking
- Being slowed down
- Trouble putting thoughts into words

Emotional (Feelings)
- Depression
- Angry outbursts and quick to anger
- Anxiety (fear, worry, or feeling nervous)
- Personality changes

These symptoms are part of the normal process of getting better. They are not signs of lasting brain damage. These symptoms are to be expected and are not a cause for concern or worry. More serious symptoms include severe forms of those listed above, decreased response to standard treatments, and seizures.

Assessment
Table 3.1 lists measures used to assess exposure to trauma.

Recovery from TBI
- Get plenty of sleep at night and rest during the day.
- Return to normal activities gradually, not all at once.
- Until you are better, avoid activities that can lead to a second brain injury such as contact or recreational sports. Remember to use helmets and safety belts to decrease your risk of having a second brain injury.
- Don't drink alcohol; it may slow your brain recovery and it puts you at risk of further injury.
- If it's harder to remember things, write them down.
- If you find you are losing important items, begin putting them in the same place all the time.

Table 3.1

Trauma Exposure Measures	Target Group	Format	# of items	Time to Administer (minutes)	Assesses DSM-IV Criterion A
Combat Exposure Scale (CES)	Adult	Self-Report	7	5	No
Evaluation of Lifetime Stressors (ELS)	Adult	Self-Report & Interview	56	60-360	Yes
Life Stressor Checklist-Revised (LSC-R)	Adult	Self-Report	30	15-30	Yes
National Women's Study Event History	Adult	Interview	17	15-30	A-1 only
Potential Stressful Events Interview (PSEI)	Adult	Interview	62	120	Yes
Stressful Life Events Screening Questionnaire (SLESQ)	Adult	Self-Report	13	10-15	No
Trauma Assessment for Adults (TAA)	Adult	Self-Report & Interview	17	10-15	A-1 only
Trauma History Screen (THS)	Adult	Self-Report	13	2-5	Yes
Trauma History Questionnaire (THQ)	Adult	Self-Report	24	10-15	A-1 only
Traumatic Events Questionnaire (TEQ)	Adult	Self-Report	13	5	A-1 only
Traumatic Life Events Questionnaire (TLEQ)	Adult	Self-Report	25	10-15	A-1 only
Trauma History Questionnaire (THQ)	Adult	Self-Report	24	10-15	Yes
Traumatic Stress Schedule (TSS)	Adult	Interview	9	5-30	A-1 only

- If you are easily distracted or having difficulty concentrating, try doing only one thing at a time in a quiet, nondistracting environment.
- If you feel irritable, then remove yourself from the situation that's irritating you or use relaxation techniques to help manage the situation. Irritability is worse when you are tired, so rest will help.
- Be patient! Healing from a brain injury takes time.

TBI SURVEILLANCE

DVBIC is tracking the numbers of service members who sustain a traumatic brain injury (TBI) in order to improve care delivery within the Department of Defense (DoD) and Department of Veterans Affairs (VA). Understanding the scope of the problem in our warrior population is essential to determine the ideal level of response at the local, regional, and national level. Specifically, improving the accuracy of statistical information helps to direct existing medical assets, develop and expand educational and clinical resources, and allows for deeper appreciation of the issue by providers and family members alike.

DVBIC began collecting surveillance data on service members who sustained a TBI in Operation Enduring Freedom (OEF)/Operation Iraqi Freedom (OIF) in 2003. Data was obtained from DVBIC-affiliated sites at military treatment facilities, VA hospitals, and civilian rehabilitation centers. In 2007, DVBIC was designated as the Office of Responsibility for the consolidation of all TBI-related incidences and prevalence information for the DoD. Today, DVBIC continues to receive new data on a monthly basis from all service branches.

A TBI classified as moderate or severe can result in short-term or long-term problems with independent function. Most TBIs are mild, and those who sustain them usually recover completely within one to three months.

One of the most common observations reported by families of service members originally not diagnosed with mTBI is that upon return from deployment, they "have changed." Classic neurological and cognitive symptoms of mTBI that should be recognized and discussed with medical professionals include

- Reduced reaction time
- Decision-making difficulties
- Decreased memory and forgetfulness

- Attention and concentration difficulties
- Confused about recent events
- Repeating of thoughts and questions
- Personality changes
- Impulsiveness
- Anger
- Sadness
- Depression
- Nervousness
- Changes in sleep patterns

Service members often overlook the symptoms of mTBI because they don't think that they are serious issues; they don't want to admit to the injury to their peers; or they don't have time to attend to these symptoms due to the fatigue and stress of a wartime environment.

While these symptoms may seem subtle to you and not obvious to others, many service members do not want to mention these symptoms to others. This is a mistake.

Awareness of the symptoms is critical for you and your family because even a doctor may not be able to recognize the subtle changes at the initial visit. Acknowledging these injuries is no longer considered a weakness, but rather a sign of strength and personal responsibility.

You must be your own advocate by knowing the symptoms for all types of brain injuries and seeking immediate medical advice if you experience any of them. The sooner these injuries are diagnosed, the more effective the treatment, and the sooner you'll be able to regain lost abilities and adapt to changes.

Symptoms of mild TBI or concussion often resolve within hours to days and almost always improve over one to three months. However, if symptoms persist without improvement, medical treatment should be sought.

CONCUSSION/mTBI SCREENING

Unlike a severe or even moderate traumatic brain injury (TBI), a concussion or mild traumatic brain injury (mTBI) may not be readily identified. Recognizing the importance of early detection, the Department of Defense (DoD) and Department of Veterans Affairs (VA) have established systemwide screening and assessment procedures to identify concussion/mTBI in service members and veterans at the soonest opportunity and through multiple points of care.

Screening for concussion/mTBI involves a quick evaluation of possible exposure to a traumatic event, including injuries that may occur during deployment, leave, or even civilian life following active duty. Clinicians work to establish if there was an alteration of consciousness (AOC) associated with the injury or traumatic event, and if the event resulted in any neurologic changes or symptoms.

In-Theater

Ideally, screening should occur immediately following the injury event or as soon as operationally feasible. The Military Acute Concussion Evaluation (MACE) is a screening tool developed by DVBIC in 2006 that allows medics/corpsmen and front-line providers to quickly measure four cognitive domains: orientation, immediate memory, concentration, and memory recall. When combined with other clinical information, the MACE score can help reveal basic cognitive performance and guide recommendations, including evacuation to a higher level of care. The MACE is currently undergoing further validation studies in a combat environment and DVBIC continues to work to ensure screening for concussion/mTBI at all levels and environments of care. The MACE alone does not diagnose concussion/mTBI.

Landstuhl Regional Medical Center

Service members with significant injuries or nonbattle medical conditions that require evacuation from theater, undergo screening for concussion/mTBI at Landstuhl Regional Medical Center (LRMC). This process identifies any history of previous brain injury (combat- or noncombat-related) and assesses for the presence or absence of current concussion/mTBI-related symptoms. Identification of newly symptomatic patients results in triage to a stateside medical facility that can more fully evaluate and, if necessary, provide treatment for concussion/mTBI.

Post-Deployment

Because concussion/mTBI is not always recognized in the combat setting, screening of active duty service members also occurs through post-deployment health assessments (PDHA). Four questions that are adapted from the *Brief Traumatic Brain Injury Survey* (BTBIS) appear on the PDHA. Positive responses on all four questions should prompt a clinician interview to more fully evaluate for concussion/mTBI.

Veterans

Screening for concussion/mTBI of veterans occurs upon entry into the Veterans Health Administration (VHA) system, using a TBI Clinical Reminder tracking system. The first step of the reminder is to identify possible Operation Enduring Freedom (OEF)/Operation Iraqi Freedom (OIF) participants based on whether date of separation from military duty or active duty status occurred after September 11, 2001. The screening for concussion/mTBI is done once for all individuals who report deployment to OEF/OIF theaters. For those who confirm OEF/OIF deployment and do not have a prior diagnosis of concussion/mTBI, the instrument proceeds using four sequential sets of questions, once again based on the *BTBIS*. Arrangements for further evaluation are offered for those who screen positive for concussion/mTBI.

It is important to realize that not all individuals whose screen is positive have a concussion/mTBI. Positive screens are always followed up by a clinical interview and examination to confirm or negate the diagnosis of a concussion/mTBI.

If you are a service member or veteran and believe you may have sustained a concussion/mTBI, DVBIC can help. Call the DVBIC at 800-870-9244 or use the "Contact Us" form to send a message online.

*   *   *

CLASSIFICATION AND NATURAL HISTORY OF TRAUMATIC BRAIN INJURIES (TBI)

Severity

Many patients and clinicians assume that the terms mild, moderate, and severe TBI refer to the severity of symptoms associated with the injury. In fact these terms refer to the nature of the injury itself. Here are the accepted definitions:

- Mild traumatic brain injury is defined as a loss or alteration of consciousness < 30 minutes, post-traumatic amnesia < 24 hours, focal neurologic deficits that may or may not be transient, and/or Glasgow Coma Score (GCS) of 13–15.

- Moderate traumatic brain injuries entail loss of consciousness > 30 minutes, post-traumatic amnesia > 24 hours, and an initial GCS 9–12.
- Severe brain injuries entail all of the moderate criteria listed above, but with a GCS < 9.

Mild TBI

About 80 percent of all TBIs in the civilian population are mild traumatic brain injuries (mTBI). The primary causes of TBIs in the civilian population are falls, motor vehicle accidents, being struck by an object, and assaults. Immediately subsequent to the initial insult, 80–100 percent of patients with mTBI will experience one or more symptoms related to their injury, such as headache, dizziness, insomnia, impaired memory, and/or lowered tolerance for noise and light. In most cases of mTBI, patients return to their previous level of function within three to six months, and it is important to reassure patients about this fact. However, some 10–15 percent of patients may go on to develop chronic post-concussive symptoms. These symptoms can be grouped into three categories: somatic (headache, tinnitus, insomnia, etc.), cognitive (memory, attention, and concentration difficulties), and emotional/behavioral (irritability, depression, anxiety, behavioral dyscontrol). Patients who have experienced mTBI are also at increased risk for psychiatric disorders compared to the general population, including depression and PTSD.

In the military population, the emerging picture is somewhat different. The primary causes of TBI in veterans of Iraq and Afghanistan are blasts, blast plus motor vehicle accidents (MVAs), MVAs alone, and gunshot wounds. Exposure to blasts is unlike other causes of mTBI and may produce different symptoms and natural history. For example, veterans seem to experience the post-concussive symptoms described above for longer than the civilian population; some studies show most will still have residual symptoms eighteen to twenty-four months after the injury. In addition, many veterans have multiple medical problems. The comorbidity of PTSD, history of mild TBI, chronic pain, and substance abuse is common and may complicate recovery from any single diagnosis. Given these special considerations, it is especially important to reassure veterans that their symptoms are time-limited and, with appropriate treatment and healthy behaviors, likely to improve.

Moderate and Severe TBI

Patients with moderate and severe brain injuries often have focal deficits and occasionally profound brain damage. However, it should be noted that the severity of the initial injury does not correlate in a linear fashion with the severity of the brain damage, and that some of these patients can make remarkable recoveries. They may need ongoing cognitive and vocational rehabilitation, case management, and pharmacological intervention to return to their highest level of function.

Diagnosis

The diagnosis of TBI, associated post-concussive symptoms, and other comorbidities such as PTSD, presents unique challenges for diagnosticians. No screening instruments available can reliably make the diagnosis; the gold standard remains an interview by a skilled clinician. The current VA screening tool is intended to initiate the evaluation process, not to definitively make a diagnosis.

Details of the original injury can be elusive. Patients with moderate and severe brain injuries often, though not always, have unequivocal evidence of the relationship of their symptoms to their injury. Patients who have experienced mTBI can be more difficult to diagnose. The brevity of the initial alteration of consciousness may cause the initial injury to go unnoticed and the patient may present some time after the original injury when details are unclear. Another factor is that these injuries can occur in chaotic circumstances, such as combat, and may be ignored in the heat of events. Clinicians may be presented with vague concerns and little relevant detail about the original injury; whenever possible, clinicians and patients should attempt to obtain supporting documentation. At minimum clinicians should elicit as detailed an injury history as possible.

Once the injury history has been established, the patient's course of recovery and remaining post-concussive symptoms should be documented. Because of the considerable symptom overlap between post-concussive symptoms and symptoms of many psychiatric and neurologic disorders, this process can be challenging. Clinicians should have a low threshold to consult available expertise when making these diagnoses.

Patients with TBI often meet criteria for PTSD on screening instruments for TBI and vice versa. Some of these positive screens may represent false positives, but many OEF/OIF veterans have experienced a mild traumatic brain injury and also have PTSD related to their combat experience.

To manage this new injury profile, the VA has initiated the Polytrauma System of Care, which treats patients with traumatic brain injury who also have experienced musculoskeletal, neurologic, and psychological trauma. Many of the most severely injured polytrauma patients are already receiving treatment at one of the four polytrauma rehabilitation centers or one of the twenty-one polytrauma network sites. Patients with milder injuries may present for treatment at other locales, including their local VAs or in their communities. Regardless of where a patient engages in treatment initially, there is no "wrong door" for treatment and the VA is working to ensure that any barriers to access are minimized.

Randomized controlled trials have demonstrated that education for the patient and family early in the course of recovery can improve outcomes in patients with TBI and help to prevent the development of other psychological problems. Unfortunately, for reasons outlined above, many patients and their families do not receive education early in the course of illness and may require intervention after symptoms have become well established. Currently, the VA encourages a recovery message when prognosis is discussed and inclusion of the family in treatment planning. Treatments for PTSD, mTBI, and other comorbidities should be symptom-focused and evidence-based in concurrence with current practice guidelines (available at www.healthquality.va.gov, VA/DoD Clinical Practice Guidelines). For example, early data shows that the treatments that have worked well in veterans with PTSD alone, such as cognitive processing therapy, prolonged exposure, or selective serotonin reuptake inhibitors (SSRIs), can also work well for veterans who have suffered a mild traumatic brain injury as well as emotional trauma. Memory aids can also be useful in this population. Patients can also benefit from occupational rehabilitation and case management, depending on the severity of their injuries. Patient should be referred to consultants, such as neurologists, neuropsychologists, and substance abuse or other specialized treatment as needed.

Given the complexity of treatment plans for these veterans, careful collaboration and coordination of care between all providers is a critical element of treatment success. The VA is exploring ways to enhance this collaboration, particularly in more community-based outpatient clinics and more rural environments.

CONCUSSIONS OR MILD TRAUMATIC BRAIN INJURY (mTBI)

Explosions that produce dangerous blast waves of high pressure rattle your brain inside your skull and can cause mTBI. Helmets cannot protect against this type of impact. In fact, 60 to 80 percent of service members who have injuries from some form of blast may have TBI.

Symptoms associated with mild TBI (or concussion) can parallel those of PTSD but also include

- Headaches or dizziness
- Vision problems
- Emotional problems, such as impatience or impulsiveness
- Trouble concentrating, making decisions, or thinking logically
- Trouble remembering things, amnesia
- Lower tolerance for lights and noise

Know that PTSD is often associated with these other conditions. However, there are effective treatments for all of these problems.

MEDICAL EVACUATION

Care for combat-wounded service members is expedited through a medical transport system which begins on the battlefield with initial life-saving treatment and continues through Combat Support Hospitals and regional medical centers, and extends into the continental United States (CONUS). There, acute care intensifies with further medical stabilization and supportive TBI care in a rapid sequence of events that ensures timely identification and treatment of injuries. The medical assets at each level of care are different, but the goal for patients with traumatic brain injury is the same: to optimize functional outcomes.

Service members sustaining moderate to severe TBI while in OEF/OIF are given emergent treatment at military facilities in theater. Once stabilized, the service member is transported to Landstuhl Regional Medical Center (LRMC) by highly skilled United States Air Force (USAF) critical care transport teams. At LRMC, there is a full complement of medical professionals that provides round the clock care to injured service members. Commonly, trauma surgery, neurosurgery, neurology, and critical care doctors and nurses implement treatment plans according to national TBI care guidelines. This may involve additional medical stabilization, imaging, and procedures.

If needed, specialists such as orthopedists, plastic surgeons, and others may be consulted.

Once all injuries are identified and initial treatment started, the patient is evacuated stateside to one of the designated inpatient TBI centers: Walter Reed Army Medical Center (WRAMC), National Naval Medical Center (NNMC), or Brooke Army Medical Center (BAMC). This cycle of evacuation can occur in as few as seventy-two hours—much more quickly than in previous conflicts, which sometimes took thirty days or more.

It is important to remember that the vast majority of brain injuries are concussions. Over 80 percent of service members sustaining a concussion will not require evacuation.

Recommendations developed by military and civilian experts, including those engaged in National Football League (NFL) and National Collegiate Athletic Association (NCAA) research, are utilized to evaluate and carefully monitor those with concussion. For those with symptoms persisting longer than two weeks, further workup may be indicated.

Once again, the initial conduit is through LRMC. The injured may undergo testing to help determine if symptoms are related to a TBI or another condition. Efforts to control certain symptoms such as headache are started. Once it is determined that additional TBI treatment is needed, arrangements are made for stateside transfer.

As with more severe injury, patients with concussion are transported via the USAF aeromedical evacuation program. Those with concussion generally do not require inpatient medical services. As a result, they may be evacuated to their home duty station if the local military treatment facility has adequate TBI resources. In the event the home duty station does not have appropriate TBI assets, the service member is transferred to a stateside location that does. Service members may be referred to medical facilities hosted by another branch of service if needed.

RETURNING TO DUTY

The vast majority of people who sustain a mild traumatic injury (mTBI)/concussion recover spontaneously without the need for specialized assessment or medical care. For others, a mTBI/concussion may have lingering effects.

After receiving a medical evaluation, service members may be given a short period of duty restrictions. This gives the brain time to heal. This is especially important for those who have a job that puts them at risk for sustaining another injury. If the service member has no symptoms and screens negative for concussion after exertional testing, then returning to duty, with education, is appropriate.

One should not return to full duty until the symptoms of concussion, like headache or dizziness are better. Other symptoms, such as eyes hurting from the light, can be managed with sunglasses. Returning to work too soon can cause a temporary worsening of symptoms if one's brain is not fully healed. Sometimes it is helpful to gradually resume one's work schedule. It is important that service members let their provider decide when it's time to return to duty.

The following considerations are important when planning one's return to work.

Schedule Considerations
- Shortened work day (e.g., 0800–1200)
- Allow for breaks when symptoms increase
- Reduced task assignments and responsibilities

Safety Considerations
- No driving
- No heavy lifting/working with machinery
- No heights if experiencing dizziness or balance deficit

DEFENSE AND VETERANS BRAIN INJURY CENTER
The Defense and Veterans Brain Injury Center (DVBIC) is a broadly based, multifaceted, multisite program created and funded by Congress as a collaboration between all branches of the Department of Defense (DoD) and Veterans Affairs (VA) with the combined designated core missions of enhancing traumatic brain injury (TBI) clinical care standards and initiatives, research, and education for the service members, veterans, and their families.

Unique Strengths
1. Unique collaboration between the VA and DoD
    a. Our program has been used as a model as senior policy leaders consider how to achieve greater partnerships between the DoD and VA for other fields of medicine.

b. Participation from all DoD components facilitates interservice coordination.

2. Multidisciplinary/Transdisciplinary approach providing objectivity
    a. The team approach allows us to always focus on objective best evidence and avoids potential influences from agenda or bias specific to a particular discipline.

3. Model of coordination and collaboration
    a. A collaborative team approach fosters greater participation from all stakeholders and avoids any complications of perceived turf or command and control.

4. Combination of clinical/educational initiatives within same organization as research initiatives
    a. This allows for clinicians to better inform pragmatic research needs and the latest research to more rapidly improve clinical care.

DEFENSE CENTERS OF EXCELLENCE (DCoE)

Mission

DCoE assesses, validates, oversees, and facilitates prevention, resilience, identification, treatment, outreach, rehabilitation, and reintegration programs for psychological health (PH) and traumatic brain injury (TBI) to ensure the Department of Defense meets the needs of the nation's military communities, warriors, and families.

Overview

Under the leadership of Army Brig. Gen. Loree K. Sutton, special assistant to the assistant secretary of defense for health affairs, DCoE was created in November 2007. DCoE is the open front door of the Department of Defense for warriors and their families needing help with PH and TBI issues, promoting the resilience, recovery, and reintegration of warriors and their families.

DCoE partners with the Department of Defense, the Department of Veterans Affairs, and a national network of military and civilian agencies, community leaders, advocacy groups, clinical experts, and academic institutions to establish best practices and quality standards for the treatment of PH and TBI. Their work is carried out across these major areas: clinical care; education and training; prevention; research; and patient, family, and community outreach.

In addition, DCoE is working to tear down the stigma that still deters some from seeking treatment for problems such as post-traumatic stress disorder and TBI with our Real Warriors Campaign.

Structure

DCoE brings together eight directorates and six component centers. Their joint goal is to maximize opportunities for warriors and families to thrive through a collaborative global network to promote resilience, recovery, and reintegration for PH and TBI.

Directorates

Clearinghouse, Outreach and Advocacy

Mission

To provide relevant information, tools, and resources for warriors, families, leaders, clinicians, and the community that empower them, support them, and strengthen their resilience, recovery, and reintegration.

Director

Cmdr. Anthony Arita

Overview

The Clearinghouse, Outreach and Advocacy Directorate provides relevant information, tools, and resources about psychological health (PH) and traumatic brain injury (TBI) to warriors, families, leaders, clinicians, and the community.

The directorate oversees the Defense Centers of Excellence for Psychological Health and Traumatic Brain Injury (DCoE) Outreach Center, which provides tools, information, and resources to military service members, veterans, their families, and others who have questions or concerns about PH and TBI. It operates 24/7. The DCoE Outreach Center is staffed by behavioral health consultants and nurses with advanced degrees and expertise in PH and TBI issues. In addition to answering questions, consultants refer callers to contact centers in the Department of Defense, other federal agencies, and outside organizations when appropriate.

Goals and Objectives
- Disseminate useful information about PH and TBI that will benefit warriors, veterans, and families.

- Disseminate information of relevance to multiple target audiences.
- Actively engage with warriors, families, caregivers, clinicians, researchers, leaders, educators, support organizations, and treatment resources to connect, share, collaborate, and coordinate to serve the needs of warrior families.
- Engage network resources to proactively identify concerns regarding the receipt, delivery, and navigation of care for wounded warriors as well as to assist in the identification and mobilization of those resources that best address those concerns.

Functional Areas

Information Clearinghouse: The directorate serves as the central source where any warrior, family member, caregiver, clinician, researcher, educator, military leader, or other interested person may obtain current information regarding PH and TBI.

Outreach: The directorate disseminates information of relevance to multiple target audiences, communicates DCoE's position as the premiere resource on PH and TBI issues and actively engages with warriors, families, caregivers, clinicians, researchers, leaders, educators, support organizations, and treatment resources to connect, share, collaborate, and coordinate to serve their needs.

Advocacy: The directorate engages network resources to proactively identify concerns regarding the receipt, delivery, and navigation of care for wounded warriors as well as to assist in the identification and mobilization of resources that best address those concerns.

Annual Gender and Ethnic Specific Conferences: The directorate is responsible for addressing the Department of Defense Task Force on Mental Health and the recommendations of the National Defense Authorization Act of 2008 to note the gender- and ethnic-specific mental health care needs of members of the armed forces. In response to this, DCoE cohosted the inaugural conference "Trauma Spectrum Disorders: The Role of Gender, Race & Other Socioeconomic Factors" in collaboration with the Department of Veterans Affairs and the National Institutes of Health. The conference was designed to improve identification and treatment of gender and race factors in traumatic stress and TBI.

Communications

Mission

The Communications Directorate informs external audiences about the work of DCoE and about issues dealing with psychological health and traumatic brain injury.

Interim Director

Ms. Catherine (Cathy) Haight

Overview

The directorate responds to queries from the news media and reaches out to the media to disseminate information. The directorate sets up media interviews with DCoE leaders and subject matter experts, and produces news releases and other material for the media. In addition, the directorate produces a monthly newsletter and operates the DCoE website and the Real Warriors Campaign website to provide information directly to external audiences. The directorate also links DCoE to other communications offices in the Department of Defense and the Department of Veterans Affairs to coordinate activities.

Goals and Objectives

To provide accurate, timely, and useful information that will benefit warriors, their families, veterans, health professionals, and the American people.

Functional Areas
- Media relations
- DCoE website
- DCoE newsletter
- Real Warriors Campaign and website

Psychological Health Clinical Standards of Care Directorate

Mission

To promote optimal clinical practice standards to maximize the psychological health (PH) of warriors and their families.

Director
   Air Force Lt. Col. Robert Wilson

Overview
   The Psychological Health Clinical Standards of Care Directorate establishes and maintains a consistent standard of excellence across the Military Health System (MHS) for PH treatment. The directorate's priority is to disseminate clinical practice guidelines with appropriate consultation and support to MHS for implementation.

Goals and Objectives
   The directorate is responsible for standardizing the use of evidence-based clinical practice guidelines and supporting state-of-the-art PH care. It also ensures consistent clinical support for patients with PH needs across the entire range of practice, from the battlefield to the MHS and beyond. This is accomplished by providing

- Clinical practice guidelines
- Consultation and site visits
- Resource support and guidance

Functional Areas
   The directorate has three primary functions:

- Clinical Practice Guidelines: In collaboration with the Department of Veterans Affairs, the directorate helps establish, refine, monitor, and renew comprehensive, joint PH clinical practice guidelines. Areas of focus include post-traumatic stress disorder, major depressive disorder, substance use disorders, acute psychosis and medically unexplained symptoms. Where no guidelines exist, the Department of Defense works with the Department of Veterans Affairs and national experts to develop them.
- Clinical Practice Consultation: The directorate provides PH consultation and visitation services to clinical programs to standardize the best PH care across the MHS and to ensure systems are in place for the seamless transition of patients with PH needs as they move through the entire spectrum of care from the battlefield, to the MHS, to the Department of Veterans Affairs, and to the civilian community.

- Clinical Practice Resource Support: The Clinical Practice Resource Support Division investigates the potential adoption of PH best practices and programs currently available at the federal, state, and community level to determine those initiatives' broad applicability for use throughout MHS. The team ensures awareness across the MHS of those evidence-based programs or best practices with the goal of standardizing care as patients move through the entire spectrum of care.

Research, Quality Assurance, Program Evaluation, and Surveillance

Mission

To improve psychological health and traumatic brain injury outcomes through research, quality programs and evaluation, and surveillance for our service members and their families.

Director

Col. Richard Ricciardi

Overview

The directorate collaborates with numerous federal and nonfederal partners and a network of other civilian agencies, community leaders, professional societies, academia, industry, and the scientific community.

Ongoing work includes planning a research program portfolio synchronization conference on psychological health (PH) and traumatic brain injury (TBI); developing a centralized research proposal database on PH and TBI; collaborating with federal and nonfederal agencies, industry, and academia to ensure a more thorough research gap analysis; leading efforts towards standardization in definitions, metrics, measures, and outcomes in PH/TBI research; participating in the clinical consortia meetings; evaluating funded PH/TBI programs; and coordinating with designated liaisons between federal and nonfederal agencies.

Goals and Objectives

The directorate has multiple goals and objectives in relation to its division missions, all supporting its overarching goal of developing and assessing evidence for improved PH and TBI care using research, surveillance, state-of-the-art treatment, and community support to improve care for America's warriors, families, leaders, and communities.

Directorate Divisions

- The Research Division facilitates scientific inquiry addressing critical areas in the fields of PH and TBI; supports and conducts scientifically meritorious, mission-relevant research to address PH issues and improve recovery of TBI patients; reviews and recommends funding of new and ongoing research protocols.
- The Quality Assurance Division develops and implements processes to conduct quality control evaluations of programs and initiatives, and serves as a resource for the organization for metric development and evaluating progress.
- The Program Evaluation Division evaluates new and ongoing funded programs that address critical areas to improve PH and decrease effects of TBI; uses empirical evidence gathered through evaluation to guide evidence-based practice and development of useful clinical practice guidelines; conducts site visits to evaluate the progress and quality of funded programs by evaluating metrics; and provides recommendations concerning continued funding or program implementation. The Surveillance Division develops and maintains awareness of patient tracking databases with a focus on PH and TBI, including registries and epidemiological and surveillance databases; participates in tracking of patient epidemiological and longitudinal data that describe the natural history of PH/TBI; uses empirical evidence to guide evidence-based practice and development of useful clinical practice guidelines; and prepares appropriate reports on PH/TBI issues.

Resilience and Prevention

Mission

Assist the Services and the Department of Defense (DoD) to optimize resilience; psychological health; and readiness for service members, leaders, units, families, support personnel, and communities.

Director (interim)

Mark Bates, Ph.D.

Overview

The Resilience and Prevention (R&P) Directorate is responsible for supporting DoD and other federal and civilian agencies' resilience and prevention efforts, programs, and initiatives. To accomplish its mission, the R&P Directorate connects with a broad range of subject matter experts and support agencies to assess and monitor needs; identify and disseminate best practices, innovative programs, and practical tools; and develop and integrate robust communities of practice.

Goals

- Facilitate a cultural shift toward a model of psychological health in the Services and DoD focused on resilience and primary prevention.
- Encourage and support ongoing multiagency and multidisciplinary collaboration among DoD leaders, federal and state agencies, medical agencies, and other support agencies that have expertise in resilience and prevention research and practices.
- Identify and disseminate best practices; innovative programs; and practical tools that empower DoD leaders, policymakers, medical agencies, and other support agencies to facilitate resilience and prevention.
- Provide needs assessments and consultation services for effectively selecting/developing, implementing, and evaluating resilience and prevention programs in various system contexts.

Functional Areas

- Facilitate a cultural shift from treatment of illness to a holistic approach for psychological health, resilience, and prevention.
- Promote resilience-building programs and practices to enhance performance and combat effectiveness; operational readiness across organizational and community systems; family and community resilience; and reintegration of service members and families, including post-deployment growth.
- Address stigma and barriers to care.
- Support prevention programs and activities targeting, but not limited to, suicide prevention, alcohol and substance abuse prevention, family maltreatment prevention, sexual assault prevention, workplace violence, and prevention of adverse stress-related mental health conditions such as post-traumatic stress disorder and depression.
- Assist in the development and maintenance of programs and services designed to support service members and their families during the process of recovery from physical and/or mental injuries.

Strategy, Plans and Programs

Mission

To foster and promote the Defense Centers of Excellence for Psychological Health and Traumatic Brain Injury strategic management efforts that help successfully prevent and treat traumatic brain injury, and to promote overall psychological health.

Acting Director

Mr. Jonathan Popa

Overview

The Strategy, Plans and Programs Directorate provides direct oversight and facilitation of the day-to-day operations of DCoE to ensure an entire spectrum of care for service members and their families. It oversees the establishment, refinement, and monitoring of all comprehensive strategies and plans for DCoE, which includes coordination of all conferences and off-site events, planning for future DCoE facilities, and the integration of DCoE with other federal agencies.

Goals and Objectives

The directorate's primary objective is to work toward enhancing the public trust and confidence in warrior and family care for psychological health and traumatic brain injury. The primary functions of the directorate are strategic planning, performance analysis and evaluation, integration and operations, and executive branch and legislative affairs.

To accomplish these objectives, the directorate facilitates integration and synergy within DCoE itself, monitoring and ensuring that all resource alignments are sound, conducts all strategic planning for the organization, assumes responsibility for performance analysis and improvement, and takes the lead on facilitating and ensuring relevant Department of Defense culture development. The directorate also promotes and coordinates external federal partnerships.

Functional Areas

The functional organization of the directorate is

- Strategic Planning: Responsible for ensuring that the strategic direction of DCoE is maintained.

- Performance Analysis and Evaluation: Responsible for the DCoE Significant Actions Report and gathering and tracking appropriate metrics.
- Integration and Operations: Responsible for tracking internal and external taskers and overseeing DCoE day-to-day operations.
- Executive Branch and Legislative Affairs: Responsible for ensuring that appropriate responses to Congress and other legislative and executive branch requests are provided in a timely fashion. The directorate also ensures that all National Defense Authorization Act requirements within DCoE are met.

Training and Education

Mission

To promote psychological health (PH) and improve traumatic brain injury (TBI) outcomes by assessing training and educational needs and identifying, integrating, developing, and disseminating effective programs for providers, service members and their families, military leaders, and communities.

Director

USPHS CAPT Gail Hamilton

Overview

The Training and Education Directorate promotes PH and improves TBI outcomes for warriors and their families. The directorate assesses the training and educational needs of varied audiences, identifies and evaluates training and educational programs to fill these needs, develops guidelines for the effective delivery of these programs, and works with partners to develop new training and education programs. The directorate also works to disseminate effective training and education programs and to expand awareness of these programs.

Training and education programs addressed by the directorate include those designed for warriors and military leaders, military families, health care and mental health care providers, and community leaders. Within this role, the directorate is responsible for identifying best practices, establishing guidelines for the delivery of PH and TBI training and education programs, and evaluating the impact of training and education programs. The directorate also serves a key role in helping to coordinate Department of Defense

(DoD) and Department of Veterans Affairs (VA) training efforts within its scope.

Goals and Objectives

The directorate aims to promote effective and efficient solutions by coordinating programs, encouraging the sharing of resources and programs across military and civilian organizations, developing standards and guidelines for these programs, and promoting the dissemination of effective PH and TBI training and education programs.

Functional Areas

The functional organization of the directorate is as follows:

- Partner Relations: The directorate promotes effective sharing of training and education program information. It also encourages partnering and collaboration as programs are developed and modified, along with the adoption of training standards and guidelines developed by the Defense Centers of Excellence for Psychological Health and Traumatic Brain Injury (DCoE). Coordination and evaluation of training/education programs requires close collaboration with various DoD programs and entities, as well as other governmental and nongovernmental agencies.
- Guidelines for Training and Education Programs: The directorate identifies, develops, and disseminates best practices and guidelines for the delivery of training and education programs in the areas of PH and TBI.
- Program Identification and Development: A key function of the directorate is to identify effective training and education programs, and to promote the development of programs where none exist. The directorate is in the process of developing a database of PH and TBI training and education resources that will allow it to become a premier resource for individuals and organizations seeking to develop and/or deliver effective training and education in the areas of PH and TBI. Where appropriate programs do not exist, the directorate works with partners to develop necessary programs. Similarly, the directorate works with partners providing training to modify existing programs to meet guidelines for training and education programs.
- Program Evaluation: Working with the Research, Quality Assurance, Program Evaluation, and Surveillance Directorate, the directorate will evaluate existing and new training and education programs.

Traumatic Brain Injury Clinical Standards of Care

Mission

To develop state-of-the-science clinical standards to maximize recovery and functioning and to provide guidance and support in the implementation of clinical tools for the benefit of all those who sustain traumatic brain injuries (TBI) in the service of our country.

Director

Katherine (Kathy) M. Helmick, M.S., R.N., CNRN, CR

Overview

The Traumatic Brain Injury Clinical Standards of Care Directorate develops clear and concise TBI clinical standards of care including clinical tools, algorithms for care, identification of best practices, and clinical practice guidelines to help optimize care. The directorate also disseminates clinical standards of care in collaboration with a number of other directorates and develops comprehensive and universal clinical practice guidelines for use by providers in the field.

In addition, the directorate identifies and makes available all relevant TBI clinical tools in a straightforward manner for use by providers in the field and collaborates with the Department of Veterans Affairs and the Department of Defense evidence-based working groups to finalize guidelines for care and ensure wide dissemination and usage.

Goals and Objectives

The overarching goal for the directorate is to create guidelines that will inform a standard of care for TBI patients across the continuum of severity and in each practice environment.

Functional Areas

The functional organization of the directorate is as follows:

- Planning: An interdisciplinary team works to gather and assess potential best practices currently available within the Military Health System (MHS). After completion of a scientific review, best practices can be prioritized to provide clear direction to the MHS to ensure state of science clinical care.
- Collaboration: Advise Health Affairs on all future iterations of the best

practices. Coordination between this directorate and the military services will ensure that best practices are disseminated and educational strategies utilized to ensure usage of best practices.

- Dissemination and Implementation: Once best practices have been established and refined, they will be distributed to the MHS. This directorate will incorporate multiple modalities of training to ensure proper understanding and utilization of these guidelines.
- Evaluation: An interdisciplinary team will conduct site visits to help provide clinical guidance to treating TBI teams throughout the MHS. The team will identify outcome measures, track patient outcomes, and assess compliance with the standards. This information will then be utilized to further improve all TBI clinical standards with the ultimate goal of providing excellent clinical TBI care.

For Warriors

DCoE is an open door to the Department of Defense for all warriors. Whether you are an active duty, National Guard or Reserve warrior, or one of our nation's veterans, DCoE can assist you in finding the answers to your questions about psychological health and traumatic brain injury.

Through partnerships with the Department of Defense, the Department of Veterans Affairs, and a national network of military and civilian agencies, community leaders, advocacy groups, clinical experts, and academic institutions, DCoE places resources in your hands to help you with your concerns. From administrative discharge, to combat stress signs and symptoms and up-to-date treatment options for psychological health concerns and traumatic brain injury, qualified health consultants are on hand 24/7 at their Outreach Center to assist you.

In addition, DCoE has launched the Real Warriors Campaign to combat the stigma associated with military service members seeking psychological health care and treatment.

NATIONAL INTREPID CENTER OF EXCELLENCE

The Intrepid Fallen Heroes Fund, a national leader in supporting the men and women of the United States Armed Forces and their families, has completed construction of the National Intrepid Center of Excellence (NICoE), an advanced facility dedicated to research, diagnosis and treatment of military personnel and veterans suffering from traumatic brain injury (TBI) and psychological health issues. The center was officially turned over to the Department of Defense in a ceremony on June 24, 2010.

NICoE is a 72,000-square-foot, two-story facility located on the Navy campus at Bethesda, Maryland, adjacent to the new Walter Reed National Military Medical Center, with close access to the Uniformed Services University, the National Institutes of Health, and the Veterans Health Administration. NICoE is designed to provide the most advanced services for advanced diagnostics; initial treatment plan and family education; introduction to therapeutic modalities; and referral and reintegration support for military personnel and veterans with TBI, post-traumatic stress, and/or complex psychological health issues. Further, NICoE will conduct research, test new protocols, and provide comprehensive training and education to patients, providers, and families while maintaining ongoing telehealth follow-up care across the country and throughout the world.

The Fisher House Foundation www.fisherhouse.org is constructing a new twenty-one-room Fisher House adjacent to NICoE to house the families of patients. Family participation in care will be a key component of the NICoE program.

Post-Traumatic Stress Disorder and Acute Stress Disorder

PTSD (POST-TRAUMATIC STRESS DISORDER)

PTSD can occur after you have been through a traumatic event. Professionals do not know why it occurs in some people and not others. But we do know PTSD is treatable.

Symptoms of PTSD

- Startling easily
- Feeling as though a certain event is happening again
- Having nightmares of terrifying events and night sweats
- Feeling distant from those you previously felt close to
- A feeling of numbness
- Feeling more aggressive or even violent
- Chronic intrusive recalling of events
- Feelings of guilt, "Why did I live and someone else died?"
- Feelings of despair
- Suffering addiction
- Contemplating suicide
- Difficulty trusting
- Feeling anxious
- Experiencing sleep problems
- Reliving the traumatic event(s) with flashbacks; these may include triggers like sounds, smells, feelings, and loud noises

- Avoiding the anniversary of the event
- Avoiding social events or places that spark memories

Reexperiencing

Bad memories of a traumatic event can come back at any time. You may feel the same terror and horror you did when the event took place. Sometimes there's a trigger: a sound, sight, or smell that causes you to relive the event.

Avoidance and Numbing

People with PTSD often go to great lengths to avoid things that might remind them of the traumatic event they endured. They also may shut themselves off emotionally in order to protect themselves from feeling pain and fear.

Hypervigilance or Increased Arousal

Those suffering from PTSD may operate on "high alert" at all times, often have very short fuses, and startle easily.

How Likely Are You to Get PTSD?

It depends on many factors, such as

- How severe the trauma was
- If you were injured
- The intensity of your reaction to the trauma
- Whether someone you were close to died or was injured
- How much your own life was in danger
- How much you felt you could not control things
- How much help and support you got following the event

STEPS TO SOLVING THE PROBLEM AND GETTING HELP

PTSD is a treatable condition. If you think you have PTSD, or just some of its reactions or symptoms (such as nightmares or racing thoughts), it's important to let your doctor or even a chaplain know. These people can help you set up other appointments as needed.

There are several steps to addressing PTSD:

- Assessment: Having a professional evaluate you with a full interview.
- Educating yourself and your family about PTSD, its symptoms, and how it can affect your life.
- Some antidepressants can relieve symptoms of PTSD. These medications do not treat the underlying cause, yet do provide some symptom relief.
- Cognitive-behavioral therapy (CBT) generally seeks to balance your thinking and help you express and cope with your emotions about the traumatic experience.

There are different types of therapy but in most you will learn

- How the problem affects you and others
- Goal setting about ways to improve your life
- New coping skills
- How to accept your thoughts and feelings, and strategies to deal with them

You are encouraged to meet with several therapists before choosing one. Finding a therapist involves learning

- What kinds of treatment each therapist offers
- What you can expect from the treatment and the therapist
- What the therapist expects of you

In 2000, the American Psychiatric Association revised the PTSD diagnostic criteria in the fourth edition of its *Diagnostic and Statistical Manual of Mental Disorders* (DSM-IV-TR). The diagnostic criteria (Criterion A–F) are specified below.

Diagnostic criteria for PTSD include a history of exposure to a traumatic event meeting two criteria and symptoms from each of three symptom clusters: intrusive recollections, avoidant/numbing symptoms, and hyperarousal symptoms. A fifth criterion concerns duration of symptoms and a sixth assesses functioning.

Criterion A: Stressor

The person has been exposed to a traumatic event in which both of the following have been present:

1. The person has experienced, witnessed, or been confronted with an event or events that involve actual or threatened death or serious injury, or a threat to the physical integrity of oneself or others.
2. The person's response involved intense fear, helplessness, or horror. Note: in children, it may be expressed instead by disorganized or agitated behavior.

Criterion B: Intrusive Recollection

The traumatic event is persistently reexperienced in at least one of the following ways:

1. Recurrent and intrusive distressing recollections of the event, including images, thoughts, or perceptions. Note: in young children, repetitive play may occur in which themes or aspects of the trauma are expressed.
2. Recurrent distressing dreams of the event. Note: in children, there may be frightening dreams without recognizable content.
3. Acting or feeling as if the traumatic event were recurring (includes a sense of reliving the experience, illusions, hallucinations, and dissociative flashback episodes, including those that occur upon awakening or when intoxicated). Note: in children, trauma-specific reenactment may occur.
4. Intense psychological distress at exposure to internal or external cues that symbolize or resemble an aspect of the traumatic event.
5. Physiologic reactivity upon exposure to internal or external cues that symbolize or resemble an aspect of the traumatic event.

Criterion C: Avoidant/Numbing

Persistent avoidance of stimuli associated with the trauma and numbing of general responsiveness (not present before the trauma), as indicated by at least three of the following:

1. Efforts to avoid thoughts, feelings, or conversations associated with the trauma
2. Efforts to avoid activities, places, or people that arouse recollections of the trauma
3. Inability to recall an important aspect of the trauma
4. Markedly diminished interest or participation in significant activities
5. Feeling of detachment or estrangement from others

6. Restricted range of affect (e.g., unable to have loving feelings)
7. Sense of foreshortened future (e.g., does not expect to have a career, marriage, children, or a normal life span)

Criterion D: Hyperarousal

Persistent symptoms of increasing arousal (not present before the trauma), indicated by at least two of the following:

1. Difficulty falling or staying asleep
2. Irritability or outbursts of anger
3. Difficulty concentrating
4. Hypervigilance
5. Exaggerated startle response

Criterion E: Duration

Duration of the disturbance (symptoms in B, C, and D) is more than one month.

Criterion F: Functional Significance

The disturbance causes clinically significant distress or impairment in social, occupational, or other important areas of functioning.
Specify if

- Acute: if duration of symptoms is less than three months
- Chronic: if duration of symptoms is three months or more

Specify if

- With or without delay onset: onset of symptoms at least six months after the stressor

COMBAT EXPOSURE SCALE (CES)

The Combat Exposure Scale (CES) is a seven-item self-report measure that assesses wartime stressors experienced by combatants. Items are rated on a five-point frequency (1 = "no" or "never" to 5 = "more than 50 times"), five-point duration (1 = "never" to 5 = "more than 6 months"), four-point frequency (1 = "no" to 4 = "more than 12 times") or four-point degree of loss (1 = "no one" to 4 = "more than 50%") scale. Respondents are asked to respond based on their exposure to various combat situations, such as firing rounds at the enemy and being on dangerous duty. The total CES score (ranging from 0 to 41) is calculated by using a sum of weighted scores, which can be classified into one of five categories of combat exposure ranging from "light" to "heavy." The CES was developed to be easily administered and scored and is useful in both research and clinical settings.

Sample Item

Were you ever surrounded by the enemy? (1 = "no" to 5 = "more than 12 times").

LIFE EVENTS CHECKLIST (LEC)

The Life Events Checklist (LEC) is a brief, seventeen-item, self-report measure designed to screen for potentially traumatic events in a respondent's lifetime. The LEC assesses exposure to sixteen events known to potentially result in PTSD or distress and includes one item assessing any other extraordinarily stressful event not captured in the first sixteen items. For each item, the respondent checks whether the event (a) happened to them personally, (b) they witnessed the event, (c) they learned about the event, (d) they are not sure if the item applies to them, and (e) the item does not apply to them.

The LEC was developed concurrently with the Clinician Administered PTSD Scale (CAPS) and is administered before the CAPS. The LEC has demonstrated adequate psychometric properties as a stand-alone assessment of traumatic exposure, particularly when evaluating consistency of events that actually happened to a respondent. The LEC has also demonstrated convergent validity with measures assessing varying levels of exposure to potentially traumatic events and psychopathology known to relate to traumatic exposure. However, the LEC does not establish that the respondent has experienced an event with sufficient severity to meet DSM-IV criteria for a traumatic exposure (Criterion A1), and it does not assess peritraumatic emotional experiences (Criterion A2).

Scoring

Items in which the respondent endorsed that the event happened to them personally receive a score of 1; all other responses receive a score of 0. Item scores are summed for a total score.

Example Item

"Natural disaster (for example, flood, hurricane, tornado, earthquake)."

WHAT IS THE DIFFERENCE BETWEEN A TRAUMA EXPOSURE MEASURE AND A PTSD MEASURE?

The purpose of a trauma exposure measure is to identify what traumatic events an individual has experienced; the purpose of a PTSD measure is to determine whether the person has PTSD symptoms related to one of the identified events. There are a variety of trauma exposure measures. Some are very broad and assess a range of negative life events as well as traumatic experiences. Others have a narrower focus and only assess Criterion A traumas that involve life threat. Similarly, there are a range of PTSD measures that can be broad enough to include symptoms other than those related to PTSD. There are also PTSD measures that are more focused on the seventeen PTSD symptoms needed to make a diagnosis. In most cases, a thorough PTSD assessment involves the use of both a broad measure and a more focused measure.

WHAT ARE THE MAIN DIFFERENCES AMONG PTSD MEASURES?

PTSD measures vary in a number of ways. There are some basic differences to consider in terms of the (1) time required to administer the measure, (2) complexity of the format, (3) reading level of the person to be assessed, and (4) cost of use. Format is an import difference among measures. Measure formats range from seventeen-item self-report measures with a single rating for each item, to structured interviews with detailed inquiries about each symptom and interviewer ratings regarding the validity of reports. Structured interviews also differ in (1) whether they have a single gate-keeping item, (2) the level of sophistication for assessing each PTSD symptom, and (3) how well the ratings reflect symptom severity and/or frequency. Although interview measures require more interviewer training and administration time, they result in a more comprehensive assessment of PTSD. The right measure for a particular purpose depends on your goal. If you want a quick screen, a self-report measure may be best. However, if you are conducting a PTSD treatment study, you may want a sensitive interview that assesses for frequency and severity of symptoms.

WHAT ARE THE MAIN DIFFERENCES AMONG TRAUMA EXPOSURE MEASURES?

Trauma exposure measures differ a great deal in length, the range of trauma types assessed, and the degree of detailed inquiry about each traumatic event. Many simply assess exposure to high-magnitude stressors that could cause traumatic stress, and others have detailed questions to follow up endorsed events. For example, one measure may have detailed questions about certain elements of an interpersonal violence experience, and another measure may only require a yes or no to the question of whether the person was exposed to a particular type of interpersonal violence. Some measures have been better validated than other measures, and some differ as to whether they assess the nature, degree, and duration of emotional responses to the stressor.

WHAT IS THE BEST MEASURE FOR ASSESSING PTSD SYMPTOMS?

Some important considerations in choosing a PTSD measure include the time required to administer the measure, the reading level of the population being sampled, whether the desire is to assess symptoms related to a single traumatic event or to assess symptoms related to multiple traumatic events (or to assess symptoms when the trauma history is unknown), the need for the assessment to correspond to DSM criteria for PTSD, the psychometric strengths and weaknesses of the measure, and the cost of using the measure. In addition, it is important that the overall complexity and language of the measure be appropriate to the population being sampled.

HOW DO I CHOOSE A MEASURE TO ASSESS TRAUMA HISTORY?

It is difficult to assess trauma history because researchers cannot firmly establish the validity of trauma-exposure measures. It is so difficult to determine whether trauma reports are accurate that the validity of even the best measures has not been very rigorously studied. That being said, it seems likely that trauma-exposure assessments will have some validity, and their clinical relevance makes them necessary.

In choosing a measure of trauma history or exposure, there is generally a trade-off between the specificity of the assessed traumatic events and the length of the assessments. Measures that query about the widest range of potentially traumatic events, and presumably yield the most accurate reports, will be the longest. Measures that are quick and easy will inquire very broadly about types of events and may "miss" idiosyncratic traumatic events. Thus, in choosing a trauma-exposure measure for research, investigators will typically need to weigh the need for a detailed trauma-exposure assessment against the time limitations for the administration. Another consideration is whether the researcher is more interested in data regarding exposure to potentially traumatic (or high-magnitude) stressors or regarding exposures that resulted in significant emotional responses. Only a few measures assess the nature, degree, and duration of emotional responses to the stressor.

HOW CAN I OBTAIN TRAUMA EXPOSURE AND PTSD ASSESSMENT MEASURES?

The American Psychological Association's ethical guidelines on psychological test instruments require advanced graduate-level training in the administration and interpretation of psychodiagnostic assessment instruments. Measures cannot be distributed to people who do not hold at least a master's degree in a clinical discipline. Graduate students must have a professor request the measure for them and use the measure under the professor's supervision.

In the Assessment section of the National Center for PTSD's website, you can find additional information about many measures, including a contact name and address for obtaining the measure. If the measure was developed by the National Center for PTSD, you can submit a request form to obtain the assessment tool.

PSYCHOLOGICAL SYMPTOMS

PTSD Symptoms

For many veterans, a diagnostic label may not be needed and may not facilitate treatment. In some circumstances, applying such a label may be counterproductive and undesirable to the veteran. A brief measure of PTSD symptoms can, however, be useful to get an idea of current PTSD symptoms a veteran might be having and to monitor treatment progress. A wide variety of brief measures of PTSD symptoms are available, and information about these (including contact information to obtain measures) can be found at www.ncptsd.va.gov.

Additional information about measures of PTSD can be found in Briere (1997), Carlson (1997), Solomon et al. (1996), and Wilson and Keane (1996).

The Posttraumatic Checklist—Civilian (PCL-C) and the Screen for Post-traumatic Stress Symptoms (SPTSS) are measures that do not key symptoms to a particular event since exposure to multiple events is common and it is not clear that people can assign symptoms to events with any accuracy or that symptoms are, in fact, uniquely associated with particular events. The PCL-C is recommended rather than the PCL-Military because it is important to assess veterans' responses to military and nonmilitary traumatic events when assessing for treatment purposes. The SPTSS may be useful with veterans who have less formal education because it has a very low reading level. It may also be useful for veterans who are reluctant to report distress because it inquires about the frequency of symptoms rather than the degree of distress they cause.

If assignment of a diagnostic label is required or desired, the Clinician Administered PTSD Scale (CAPS) (Weathers, Keane, & Davidson, 2001) can be used. Detailed information about this structured interview and how to obtain it are available at www.ncptsd.va.gov.

Dissociation

Dissociative symptoms are very common in trauma survivors, and they may not be spontaneously reported. The Trauma-Related Dissociation Scale (Carlson & Waelde, 2000) is a measure of dissociation.

Depression

Depression is a very common comorbid condition in those with posttraumatic disorders. It may be secondary to PTSD or associated with aspects of traumatic events such as losses. The Beck Depression Inventory (BDI)—Short Form is a common brief measure of depression (Beck & Steer, 2000). This measure is also available for computerized administration via the Decentralized Hospital Computer Program (DHCP) at VA Medical Centers.

Traumatic Grief

Screen for Complicated Grief is a brief measure of symptoms of traumatic grief.

Alcohol Use

Substance use is a common problem for those with PTSD, particularly alcohol abuse and dependence. The AUDIT (Goldman, Brown, & Christiansen, 2000) is a screen for alcohol use.

Anger

Anger is a frequent problem for trauma survivors, and outbursts of anger are a symptom of PTSD. If a veteran reports problems with anger, detailed assessment of that area may be useful.

The State-Trait Anger Expression Inventory (STAX-I) is measure of anger and how it is expressed (Spielberger, 1988). This measure may be useful to assess vets, although it is important to note that it is not ideal to assess recent, post-trauma anger because its trait form assesses both pre-trauma and post-trauma anger and its state form assesses feelings at the time of the assessment (which may not be representative of the entire post-trauma period).

Guilt and Shame

Guilt and shame are frequently issues for trauma survivors who feel distressed over what they did or did not do at the time of trauma. Kubany et al. (1995) have developed a measure of guilt that may be useful to assess those with clinical issues in that domain.

Relevant History

Exposure to Potentially Traumatic Events

Because exposure to previous traumatic stressors may affect response to traumatic stressors experienced in the military, it is important to broadly assess exposure to traumatic stressors. The Trauma History Screen (Carlson, 2002) is a brief assessment tool that can be used for that purpose.

Selected scales within the Deployment Risk and Resilience Inventory (DRRI; King, King, & Vogt, 2003) may be used as a vehicle to identify particular combat and other high-magnitude and threatening experiences that were potentially traumatic. Because the level of nontraumatic stressors and the overall context in which exposure to traumatic stressors occurs may affect the response to high-magnitude stressors, it is important to assess these elements. Several scales from the DRRI (e.g., concerns about life and family disruptions, difficult living and working environment, war-zone social support) may prove useful to gain a broader profile of the deployment experience. Copies of the individual DRRI measures, scoring guides, and a full manual describing instrument development may be obtained by contacting dawne.vogt@med.va.gov.

For Women Veterans

Because women who serve in the military may be exposed to a number of traumatic stressors that are not assessed in combat measures, specific assessment of military stressors is often helpful for women veterans. The Life Stressors Checklist (Wolfe & Kimerling, 1997) was developed for this purpose.

OTHER PTSD TREATMENT OPTIONS

As a new generation of service members returns from deployment, the Department of Defense (DoD) is faced with the challenge of identifying the most effective methods of treatment to address post-traumatic stress disorder (PTSD). Prevalence estimates of PTSD symptoms based on self-report surveys among OEF/OIF warriors vary, but it has clearly been shown to be a significant problem, especially for those exposed to sustained ground combat.[1]

There are several treatment options that health professionals and clinicians can use to effectively treat service members with PTSD. Since there are a number of factors to consider in treating PTSD (e.g., access to services, availability, safety, patient preferences, etc.), it is important to understand the different types of treatments available to service members.

Prevention

As with all conditions, successful prevention of PTSD would be more desirable than even the most effective treatment. To the extent that traumatic experiences themselves may be avoided, PTSD may sometimes be prevented. In the immediate aftermath of traumatic exposure, preventive interventions are available, including psychoeducation, grief counseling and prophylactic medication. Although some of these are promising, none has yet been proven to prevent PTSD.

A number of early interventions have been utilized for the prevention of PTSD. The most promising of these are public health or population-based interventions informed by the evidence supporting cognitive-behavioral therapy (CBT) for PTSD. Psychological first aid is one example of a promising early intervention. Similarly, a growing number of well-controlled studies have demonstrated the effectiveness of CBT and exposure-based treatments as early interventions. Interventions such as these may decrease the likelihood of persons developing PTSD after traumatic exposures; however, additional research is needed to demonstrate this with certainty. Critical Incident

Stress Debriefing (CISD) has been shown to be ineffective for the prevention of PTSD following trauma exposure and is not recommended in the current VA/DoD clinical practice guideline.

Counseling

The main treatments for people with PTSD are counseling (known as "talk" therapy or psychotherapy), medications, or both. Although there are a number of treatment options for PTSD, and patient response to treatment varies, some treatments have been shown to have more benefit in general.

Cognitive-behavioral therapy (CBT) is one type of counseling. With CBT, a therapist helps the service member dealing with PTSD understand and change how thoughts and beliefs about the trauma, and about the world, cause stress and maintain current symptoms. Table 4.1 describes several types of CBT.

CBT has been shown to be successful in treating PTSD in a number of well-controlled studies.[2] However, there are a handful of service members for whom certain interventions may be inappropriate or for whom other treatment problems (e.g., co-occurring conditions) may also need to be addressed. Visit the Cautions Regarding Cognitive-Behavioral Interventions Provided within a Month of Trauma fact sheet from the VA National Center for PTSD for more information. In addition to cognitive-behavioral therapy, eye movement desensitization and reprocessing (EMDR) is another type of therapy for PTSD. EMDR uses a combination of talk therapy with specific eye movements. Evidence of its effectiveness is mixed. In general, it appears that the talk therapy component is helpful, but most evidence suggests that the eye movement component does not add much, if any, benefit. As with other kinds of counseling, the general psychotherapy component of EMDR can help change the reactions to memories service members experience as a result of their trauma(s).

Additional Types of Counseling

In addition to the treatments described above, other types of counseling may be helpful in treating PTSD.

Through group therapy, service members can talk about their trauma or learn skills to manage symptoms of PTSD (depending on the focus of the group). Many groups are effective and popular among those who have had similar traumatic experiences. Group therapy can help those with PTSD by

Table 4.1

Type of CBT	Overview/Components	Goal
Prolonged Exposure Therapy	• Imaginal exposure: Repeated and prolonged recounting of the traumatic experience • In vivo exposure: Systematic confrontation of trauma-related situations that are feared and avoided, despite being safe	Increase emotional processing of the traumatic event so that memories or situations no longer result in • Anxious arousal to trauma • Escape and avoidance behaviors
Cognitive Therapy	• Modify the relationships between thoughts and feelings • Identify and challenge inaccurate or extreme negative thoughts • Develop alternative, more logical or helpful thoughts	• Help the individual recognize and adjust trauma-related thoughts and beliefs • Help the individual modify his or her appraisals of self and the world
Cognitive Processing Therapy	Includes elements of Cognitive Therapy and Prolonged Exposure Therapy, including • Identifying and challenging problematic thoughts and beliefs (as noted above) • Particular attention is paid to "stuck points": feelings, beliefs, and thoughts that stem from the traumatic events or are hard to accept • Writing and reading aloud a detailed account of the traumatic event	• Help the individual modify beliefs about safety, trust, power/control, esteem, and intimacy • Help the individual identify and modify "stuck points"
Stress Inoculation Training	• Provide a variety of coping skills that are useful in managing anxiety, including muscle relaxation, breathing retraining, and role playing, as well as cognitive techniques, such as guided self-talk • May also include graduated in vivo exposure	• Decrease avoidance and anxious responding related to the trauma-related memories, thoughts and feelings

giving them a chance to share their stories with others, feel more comfortable talking about their own trauma, and by connecting with others who have experienced similar problems or feelings. Some types of cognitive-behavioral therapy can also be provided in a group setting.

Family and couples therapy are methods of counseling that include the service member's family members. A therapist helps all of those involved communicate, maintain good relationships, and cope with challenging emotions.[3] PTSD can sometimes have a significant negative impact on relationships, making this mode of therapy particularly helpful in some cases.

Pharmacological Approaches

Selective serotonin reuptake inhibitors (SSRIs) are a type of antidepressant medication. SSRIs include citalopram (Celexa), fluoxetine (Prozac), paroxetine (Paxil), fluvoxamine (Luvox), and sertraline (Zoloft). Many, if not most, patients with PTSD will achieve some symptom relief with an SSRI, although the evidence of effectiveness is less convincing in combat PTSD compared to PTSD due to other traumas. Additional medications have been used for specific symptoms with some success. See the VA/DoD PTSD Clinical Practice Guidelines (CPGs) at www.healthquality.va.gov/ for additional information.

Prazosin may be promising for trauma-related nightmares. In addition, short-term use of a medication for sleep can be helpful for those who have significant difficulty sleeping immediately after a traumatic event. Longer-term use of sedative/hypnotic medications, such as benzodiazepines, however, has not been shown to be of benefit, and there is some evidence that long-term use of benzodiazepines in PTSD may interfere with psychotherapy.

Complementary and Alternative Medicine

Complementary and alternative medicine (CAM) approaches to the treatment of many medical and mental health diagnoses, including PTSD, are in use; the research base to support their effectiveness is improving, but not complete. Acupuncture, a component of traditional Chinese medicine, has been examined for PTSD in a limited number of small randomized controlled trials (RCTs). Although early results are promising, replication of these results in larger studies is needed. Yoga Nidra, a relaxation and meditative form of yoga, has also been used as an adjunctive treatment for PTSD. Formal studies demonstrating its effectiveness for PTSD are currently being conducted, and further research is needed on Yoga Nidra for PTSD before its effectiveness can be commented on. Herbal or dietary supplements have also been used for the treatment of PTSD. Although there have been some studies of their effectiveness, the results of these small RCTs provide insufficient evidence to draw firm conclusions about their effectiveness for PTSD. In addition, the quality and purity of herbals and dietary supplements available in the United States vary widely, further complicating their use. Revisions of the VA/DoD CPGs are currently under way to include a comprehensive review of the evidence for all treatments, including CAM.

GUIDELINES AND RESOURCES

PTSD 101, made available by the VA's National Center for PTSD, is a web-based educational resource that is designed for practitioners who provide services to military men and women and their families as they recover from combat stress or other traumatic events.

Additional Resources

Center for the Study of Traumatic Stress

PTSD 101

Traumatic Grief: Symptomatology and Treatment for the Iraq War Veteran

PTSD in Iraq War Veterans: Implications for Primary Care

Treatment of Medical Casualty Evacuees

Traumatic Brain Injury and PTSD

Psychological First Aid: Field Operations Guide—SAMHSA

Readiness to Change in PTSD Treatment (video)

RESPECT-Mil Primary Care Physician's Manual

NACBT-Cognitive-Behavioral Therapy

Deployment Health Clinical Center—Medications

International Society for Traumatic Stress Studies—Treatment Guidelines

ASSESSMENT AND TREATMENT OF ANGER IN COMBAT-RELATED PTSD

Casey T. Taft, Ph.D. and Barbara L. Niles, Ph.D.

Veterans of Operation Iraqi Freedom who suffer from symptoms of PTSD are likely to have difficulties with anger regulation given the centrality of anger in the human survival response.

Research among military veterans has consistently shown that those with PTSD are higher in anger, hostility, aggression, general violence, and relationship violence and abuse than those without the disorder (e.g., Jordan et al., 1992). "Irritability and outbursts of anger" represent one of the diagnostic criteria for PTSD and can have a debilitating impact across several domains. Anger dysregulation typically has a deleterious impact on the veteran's relationships with family members and other loved ones, and may significantly interfere with other social and occupational functioning. These interpersonal difficulties may have a profound negative effect on the veteran's social support network, which places him or her at risk for PTSD exacerbation, and possibly for cardiovascular disease and other health problems that have been associated with anger, hostility, and PTSD. Angry outbursts may also place the veteran at risk for legal problems and may lead to severe consequences for those who are exposed to these outbursts.

Although little theory or research explicates the role of PTSD with respect to anger, one important theory for anger problems among veterans with PTSD emphasizes the role of context-inappropriate activation of cognitive processes related to a "survival mode" of functioning (Chemtob, Novaco, Hamada, Gross, & Smith, 1997).

This response includes heightened arousal, a hostile appraisal of events, a loss in the ability to engage in self-monitoring or other inhibitory processes, and resulting behavior produced to respond to this perceived severe threat. These processes lead the veteran to see threats in the civilian environment that do not objectively pose any significant danger, and he or she may respond in an aggressive manner to such threats. This "survival mode," while adaptive in combat situations, typically becomes maladaptive when the individual interacts with his or her environment in civilian life. Therefore, in therapy with this population, an important treatment target often involves the detection of cognitive biases with respect to environmental threats and the detection of disconfirming evidence. This sense of heightened threat may be particularly acute among individuals who served in Operation Iraqi Freedom because the enemy was not always clearly defined and military personnel were forced to be vigilant to attack at all times.

Assessment of Anger and Related Constructs

Anger, hostility, and aggression are typically assessed via self-report questionnaire measures of these constructs. Two of the most widely used measures are the Buss Durkee Hostility Inventory (BDHI; Buss & Durkee, 1957) and the State-Trait Anger Expression Inventory (STAX-I; Spielberger, 1988).

The BDHI (Buss & Durkee, 1957) is the most widely used measure of hostility. The measure consists of seventy-five true-false items, and eight subscales: Assault, Indirect Hostility, Verbal Hostility, Irritability, Negativism, Resentment, Suspicion, and Guilt. The measure has received criticism based on methodological grounds (e.g., low predictive validity, poor reliability), and was recently revised by Buss and Perry (1992). The new measure, called the Aggression Questionnaire, consists of twenty-nine items that are rated on a five-point Likert scale. An advantage of this measure is that it taps not only anger, but also the related constructs of hostility and aggression. Specifically, subscales include Anger, Hostility, Verbal Aggression, and Physical Aggression. This new measure and its subscales have been found to exhibit good psychometric properties.

The STAX-I (Spielberger, 1988) is a forty-four-item measure that consists of subscales tapping State Anger, Trait Anger, and Anger Expression. This measure has some benefits over other existing anger measures. First, it distinguishes state anger and trait anger, and further distinguishes between the experience of anger and the expression of anger. Subscales can also be derived to assess whether individuals tend to keep in their anger (Anger-In), or express their anger openly (Anger-Out), or whether individuals effectively control and reduce their feelings of anger (Anger Control). These distinctions may be particularly important with veterans returning from Iraq. As described in the sections that follow, these men and women are likely to have problems with holding anger in and/or acting outwardly aggressive, and may vacillate between these two extremes. Therefore, this fine-grained assessment of the individual's anger expression style may assist in treatment planning.

Challenges for Anger Interventions

Veterans with PTSD frequently report that anger is one of their most troublesome problems, and anger often prompts their treatment entry. However, evidence suggests that anger and violence are often the precipitants for early termination from treatment, and higher anger levels are associated with poorer outcomes in treatment for PTSD more generally. This section highlights a number of important challenges for intervention with PTSD-positive veterans who have anger regulation problems.

For many who have served in Operation Iraqi Freedom, the thought of openly discussing their difficulties with anger and finding alternatives to threatening or intimidating responses to everyday frustrations may seem to have life-threatening implications. The individual's anger and aggressive behavior may have been very functional in the military and in combat situations and may serve as a valuable source of self-esteem. Therefore, attempts to change an anger response may be met with considerable resistance. The advantages or disadvantages of the individual's anger expression style should be discussed in order to move him or her in the direction of behavior change.

Generally, veterans will list several serious negative consequences of their anger regulation problems and few benefits that cannot be achieved by other, more appropriate means. Therefore, discussion of the "pros" and "cons" of their anger style often serves as a powerful technique for enhancing motivation.

Veterans may resist attempts to participate in treatment for anger problems because they may associate authority figures with distrust. Angry veterans may also become impatient during the treatment process due to their desire to gain relief from their anger problems and their general heightened level of hostility and frustration. They may become easily frustrated when changes do not immediately occur as a result of therapy, and may become hostile or otherwise resistant to therapy. It is important that the treatment provider fully discusses each of these concerns with the veteran, who should be encouraged to appropriately communicate his or her concerns during the course of treatment. Given the difficulty of the therapeutic endeavor, it is critical that the provider and veteran establish and maintain a positive therapeutic relationship. The provider should also be very clear in his or her expectations for treatment. He or she should stress to the veteran that one's anger expression style is learned, and the skills required to alter anger patterns will take time to master.

Several psychiatric problems tend to be highly comorbid with PTSD, such as depression and substance abuse. These problems also pose potential barriers for effective treatment of anger problems among those with PTSD. In addition, veterans with PTSD are more likely to suffer from physical health problems, and often suffer from severe social and occupational impairments. These factors serve to increase stress and ameliorate emotional and tangible resources for the veteran, placing him or her at additional risk for anger dysregulation and violence perpetration. Further, these factors may lead to a reduced ability to make use of treatment for anger problems. The veteran's capacity to marshal the cognitive resources to do the work of therapy (e.g., participate in self-monitoring exercises or practice communication skills) and to comply with the demands of treatment may be compromised. The treatment provider, therefore, must fully assess for comorbid problems and their impact on both the veteran's anger and his or her compliance with therapy, and should ensure that the veteran receives appropriate treatment for comorbid problems. For example, substance abuse must be addressed due to its disinhibiting effects with respect to anger and aggression.

Anger Management Intervention

Most PTSD treatment programs recommend and offer varied modalities and formats for the treatment of anger problems among veterans. Programs typically offer individual and group therapies, and cognitive-behavioral treatments for anger appear to be the most common.

Increasingly, PTSD programs are utilizing manualized or standardized group treatments for anger treatment, and there is some research evidence for the effectiveness of such treatments (Chemtob, Novaco, Hamada, Gross & Smith, 1997). Below, we briefly outline session content derived from a twelve-week standardized cognitive-behavioral group treatment for anger among veterans with PTSD.

Although this material derives from a group treatment approach, the issues raised are relevant for other therapy formats and modalities.

Overview of the Treatment

The goal of our anger management group is for veterans to learn to understand and to better regulate their anger responses through greater awareness of their anger triggers and an application of constructive anger management strategies. Additionally, veterans' appraisals of threat in their environment and daily experience of anger are targeted as they learn to prepare back-up responses (e.g., time-outs, relaxation, cognitive restructuring, ventilation, and positive distraction). Each session consists of group discussions and skills-building exercises. We have found that each group of veterans will present with special needs and the sessions should be adapted accordingly. Group leaders vary their coverage of the material to best complement the unique needs of their group, and make efforts to encourage group cohesion and a safe and supportive group atmosphere.

The first two sessions of group are devoted to orienting the veterans to treatment, discussing treatment goals and expectations of therapy, enhancing motivation to work on anger management, and providing psychoeducation on the anger response and the impact of PTSD on anger. Sessions 3 through 7 are devoted to self-monitoring exercises so that the veteran may better understand his or her anger response, developing an understanding of the distinction between different forms of anger expression, learning to use relaxation strategies for managing anger, and exploring motivational issues that may be impeding progress. The remaining sessions focus on communication skills and learning to communicate assertively, barriers to anger management posed by comorbid problems, and wrapping up.

Setting Treatment Goals and Exploring Motivation

As discussed previously, it is extremely important that veterans with PTSD set realistic and attainable goals with respect to anger management, in order to prevent frustration with the therapy process and to reduce dropout. Both at the outset of therapy and throughout the course of treatment, motivational issues and barriers to successful barrier change should be explored. Also as discussed, for many veterans, anger dysregulation and aggressive behavior have served several adaptive functions, and anger expression styles may have been learned and reinforced throughout the life of the veteran.

Therefore, discussions should center not only on the negative consequences of anger dyscontrol, but also on those factors that are maintaining these maladaptive behaviors, as well as more adaptive behaviors that may serve as substitutes for identified problematic behaviors.

Psychoeducation on Anger and PTSD

In order for veterans to better understand their anger dysregulation and to develop skills to better manage anger, it is important that they understand the constructs of anger and PTSD, and how the two are related. Veterans have often been noted to experience considerable relief upon the realization that their anger problems are directly related to their PTSD symptoms, and that others are experiencing the same difficulties. In addition to providing definitions of anger and PTSD, group leaders discuss the different components of the anger response (thoughts, emotions, physiology, and behaviors), and how these components are interrelated and negatively affected by PTSD. Further, it should be stressed that the goal of treatment is not to eliminate anger completely, since the anger response is a survival response that, when communicated in a constructive manner, can be very useful and healthy. Therefore, group leaders stress that the goal of anger treatment is to learn to manage anger better and express anger in an assertive manner.

Self-monitoring

In order for veterans to learn new ways of handling their anger, they must first come to recognize when they are beginning to get angry, and recognize the thoughts and feelings associated with anger, as well as changes in their physiology. Many veterans returning from the war in Iraq may find this to be a difficult task, as their anger responses may be conditioned to respond immediately to the slightest risk of threat in their environment. That is, they may view their anger and aggression occurring instantly upon exposure to a perceived threat. However, upon completion of self-monitoring homework and in-group exercises, most group members will learn to identify signs of anger (e.g., heart racing, thoughts of revenge, feelings of betrayal) prior to an angry outburst. It is very important for veterans to develop this recognition as early as possible in the anger cycle, so that they may take active steps to avoid escalation to aggression (e.g., by taking a time-out, using relaxation strategies, etc.). Self-monitoring exercises also provide important information regarding the veteran's perceptions of threat in his or her environment, which may be appropriately challenged in the therapy context.

Assertiveness Training

Many veterans have learned to respond to threats or other potentially anger-provoking stimuli either in an aggressive manner (e.g., physical or verbal assaults) or in a passive manner. Veterans may fear their own aggressive impulses and may lack self-efficacy with respect to controlling their anger, and therefore, they are more likely to "stuff" their anger and avoid conflict altogether. Not surprisingly, this overly passive behavior often leads to feelings of resentment and a failure to resolve problems, which in turn, leads to a higher likelihood of subsequent aggressive behavior. Therefore, considerable time in treatment is devoted to making the distinctions clear between passive, aggressive, and assertive behavior, and group members are encouraged to generate and practice assertive responses to a variety of situations.

Stress Management

In combating anger regulation problems, stress management interventions are critical to reduce the heightened physiological arousal, anxiety, depression, and other comorbid problems that accompany PTSD and contribute to anger problems. In our protocol, we implement an anger arousal exercise followed by a breathing-focused relaxation exercise to assist the veteran in becoming more aware of how thoughts are related to anger arousal and how relaxation exercises can assist in defusing the anger response. The aim is to assist the veteran in creating an early warning system that will help him or her recognize and cope with anger before it escalates to aggressive behavior. In addition to the implementation of relaxation strategies, several other stress management strategies are discussed and emphasized (e.g., self-care strategies, cognitive strategies) and the importance of social support in managing anger (e.g., talking with a friend or family member when angry) is stressed throughout the course of treatment.

Communication Skills Training

Anger dysregulation often results from a failure to communicate effectively and assertively, and likewise, heightened anger and PTSD hinder communication. In our group treatment for anger problems, we cover several communication strategies (e.g., active listening, the "sandwich technique") and tips (e.g., using "I statements," paraphrasing, refraining from blaming or using threatening language) for effective communication. In this regard, is important to emphasize both verbal and nonverbal communication, as veterans with PTSD often unknowingly use threatening or intimidating looks or gestures to maintain a safe distance from others.

*   *   *

Acute Stress Disorder (ASD)

How Is ASD Diagnosed?

Because ASD is a relatively new diagnosis, there are few well-established and empirically validated measures to assess it. Although a comprehensive review of assessment measures is beyond the scope of this discussion, the tools with the strongest psychometric properties are described below:

- The Acute Stress Disorder Interview (ASDI) is the only structured clinical interview that has been validated against DSM-IV criteria for ASD. It appears to meet standard criteria for internal consistency, test-retest reliability, and construct validity. The interview was validated by comparing it with independent diagnostic decisions made by clinicians with experience in diagnosing both ASD and PTSD.

- The Acute Stress Disorder Scale (ASDS) is a self-report measure of ASD symptoms that correlates highly with symptom clusters on the ASDI. It has good internal consistency, test-retest reliability, and construct validity. Both scales may be found in Bryant and Harvey's text on ASD.

Are There Effective Treatments for ASD?

Cognitive-Behavioral Interventions

At present, cognitive-behavioral interventions during the acute aftermath of trauma have yielded the most consistently positive results in terms of preventing subsequent posttraumatic psychopathology. Four out of five randomized clinical trials (RCTs) related to early cognitive-behavioral interventions during the acute aftermath of trauma found that the cognitive-behavioral therapy (CBT) group experienced a greater reduction of PTSD symptoms than comparison groups. One of the RCTs did not find this to be true. The study by Brom et al. (1993) found that all three active conditions (desensitization, hypnotherapy, and psychodynamic therapy) yielded equal improvement relative to the waitlist control group. However, the Brom et al. study lacked a treatment adherence measure so it is unclear whether the CBT intervention was implemented in a standardized manner relative to other studies of CBT.

A different controlled (but not randomized) comparison of a CBT versus an assessment-only course of action in the acute phase post-trauma found fewer PTSD symptoms in the CBT group at a five-and-a-half-month follow-up.

Bryant and colleagues have conducted the only studies that specifically assessed and treated ASD. They have shown that a brief cognitive-behavioral treatment may not only ameliorate ASD, but it may also prevent the subsequent development of PTSD. Approximately ten days after exposure to an MVA, industrial accident, or nonsexual assault, Bryant and colleagues randomly assigned those with ASD to five individual, one-and-a-half-hour sessions of either a cognitive-behavioral treatment or a supportive counseling control condition. They found that fewer CBT subjects met criteria for PTSD post-treatment and six months later. In the 1999 study, Bryant and colleagues compared two different individual CBT approaches (prolonged exposure plus anxiety management and prolonged exposure alone) to a supportive counseling intervention. They found that both CBT groups showed significantly greater reductions in PTSD symptom severity compared to the supportive counseling group. (Please see Bryant and Harvey's text (2000) for a detailed description of their cognitive-behavioral intervention for ASD.)

Psychological Debriefing?

Psychological debriefing is an early intervention that was originally developed for rescue workers that has been more widely applied in the acute aftermath of potentially traumatic events. However, RCTs of debriefing have yielded inconsistent findings in terms of its efficacy. A review of the literature on debriefing RCTs concluded that there is little evidence to support the continued use of debriefing with acutely traumatized individuals. Mitchell and Everly (2000), the originators of the debriefing model, have made the cogent argument that most of the debriefing RCTs to date have studied only one component (debriefing) of the longer-term and more comprehensive Critical Incident Stress Management model. It is possible that this more comprehensive intervention would prove efficacious, but to date no RCTs have been conducted using the full intervention.

NOTES

1. Smith, T.C. (2007). New onset and persistent symptoms of post-traumatic stress disorder self reported after deployment and combat exposures: Prospective population based US military cohort study. *British Medical Journal*; Hoge, C.W., Castro, C.A., Messer, S.C., McGurk, D., Cotting, D.I., Koffman, R.L. (2004). Combat duty in Iraq and Afghanistan, mental health problems, and barriers to care. *New England Journal of Medicine*; Hoge, C.W., Terhakopian, A., Castro, C.A., Messer, S.C., Engel, C.C. (2007). Association of posttraumatic stress disorder with somatic symptoms, health care visits, and absenteeism among Iraq war veterans. *American Journal of Psychiatry.*

2. Cognitive processing therapy for veterans with military related post traumatic stress disorder. Retrieved August 18, 2009, from www.thesafenetwork.org/Images/cog proc therapy and ptsd.pdf.

3. Benedek, D., et. al. (2009). Guideline watch (March 2009): Practice guideline for the treatment of patients with acute stress disorder and posttraumatic stress disorder. *Focus.*

From a Medical Perspective

PSYCHIATRIC CARE IN THE MILITARY TREATMENT SYSTEM

After first being air evacuated (AE) from the theater of war to Landstuhl Regional Medical Center in Germany, most patients may be sent to one of four stateside medical center regions. These include Walter Reed Army Medical Center (WRAMC), Washington D.C.; Dwight D. Eisenhower Army Medical Center, Fort Gordon, Georgia; Madigan Army Medical Center, Fort Lewis, Washington; and Brooke Army Medical Center, Fort Sam, Houston, Texas. With some exceptions, this process is the same for army, navy, and air force personnel being air evacuated from the war zone.

Patients who are AE but only require routine outpatient care are sent to the medical center closest to the site from which they were initially mobilized. On arrival at the medical center, patients are triaged to ensure that outpatient care is, in fact, appropriate. They are then processed through the region's Deployment Health Clinical Center (DHCC) for further medical screening, and referred for treatment near their mobilization sites. While at the demobilization site, they continue to receive treatment and are evaluated for appropriate disposition. Veterans who require more intensive services are assigned to the medical center's Medical Holding Company and treated there.

Veterans who do not meet medical fitness standards are referred to a Medical Evaluation Board (MEB). Those who are determined unsuitable either because of preexisting condition or personality disorder are administratively separated. Those who are fit for duty with minor limitations are retained at the demobilization site for the remainder of their current term of service (reserve component) or released to their home duty station (active component).

A veteran requiring routine outpatient care usually remains at each echelon level hospital for seven to ten days until reaching his or her final destination. Due to time constraints, treatment is generally focused on acute symptom relief and supportive therapy. Case management serves to identify appropriate resources to provide definitive treatments, when required.

Treatment availability varies from one site to the next. If a treatment modality is required and it is not offered at the final destination, consideration is given to the potential benefit of keeping a patient at the medical center for a longer period. More often than not, the military patient wishes to return home and does not want to delay the process any more than is necessary. In these cases, psychoeducation focuses on the early identification of symptoms and the importance of self-referral for rapid mental health intervention.

Any military patients requiring a MEB or who may require intensive outpatient care or inpatient care are air evacuated to a medical center. While programs vary with respect to available services, the process at WRAMC serves as an example of treatment practices at the medical center level.

WRAMC offers several levels of mental health treatment. Upon arrival the on-call psychiatrist screens all air evacuated patients for acute symptoms that might necessitate hospitalization. Any patient air evacuated as an inpatient is admitted to the hospital and is continued in inpatient care until clinical safety is determined. During the course of the inpatient admission a comprehensive assessment is performed and treatment initiated.

Army personnel requiring a Medical Evaluation Board remain at Walter Reed and are assigned to the Medical Holding Company. Air Force and Navy personnel undergoing a MEB may be followed in the WRAMC Continuity Service within the partial hospitalization program until stabilized and ready for further disposition. Navy personnel undergoing a MEB are usually assigned to a medical holding unit near their home of record. Air Force personnel undergoing a Medical Evaluation Board typically are returned to their unit. Inpatients with more severe illnesses and who are refractory to treatment may be discharged directly from the service to a VA inpatient ward near their home.

Outpatient follow-up is variable at all locations. Most if not all locations will have some form of treatment available. The WRAMC mental health services are presented as a model of the process most mental health patients may experience in one form or another.

The WRAMC Continuity Service offers several levels of care to include intensive outpatient services (defined as patients who require more than once-weekly therapy) and partial hospitalization (defined as daily treatment of at least three hours each day). Partial hospitalization serves as a step-down unit for inpatients transitioning to outpatient care or a step-up unit for outpatients who need more care than can be given in a routine outpatient setting. Treatment modalities include group, individual, medication management, family and couples therapies as well as command consultations. Services are geared toward the needs of the patient. Daily war zone stress–related groups and individual therapies are available. Continuity Service also provides ongoing mental health treatment and case management for patients assigned to the Medical Holding Company to ensure effective psychiatric monitoring through the MEB process.

All Army mental health outpatients, whether they arrive as outpatients or are subsequently discharged from the inpatient service, are case managed by the Continuity Service until they leave WRAMC. This ensures continuity of care and provides a resource that the patient can use during the time spent at WRAMC. Those identified as primary mental health patients are monitored by the Continuity Service even if they are getting treatment on a different clinical service at WRAMC.

The Behavioral Health Service is an outpatient treatment resource for "routine" ambulatory care, acute assessments, and liaison with military patients' units in the region. Treatments offered include individual and group therapies and medication management. Patient referrals come from the air evacuation system, local units, and other medical specialties. The patient completes a comprehensive workup and an appropriate treatment plan is generated. Like the Inpatient and Continuity Service this can include return to duty, administrative separations, or referral to a MEB. Psychiatry Consultation and Liaison Service (PCLS) screens all hospitalized wounded in action (WIA) service members and most non-battle injury (NBI) members. Disease non-battle injury (DNBI) patients are also regularly evaluated by PCLS when requested through routine consultation. A mental health screening is performed on every patient admitted from the war zone and consists of a diagnostic interview and psychoeducation about combat stress, ASD, and PTSD. Service members needing further psychiatric care are referred for treatment with PCLS, Continuity Services, or Behavioral Health as needed.

Patients requiring administrative separation or a Medical Evaluation Board may be delayed in separation from the service for several months. The types of treatments available throughout the DoD vary depending upon location and available resources. The patients may receive therapy from any of the modalities discussed above and may be involved in various treatment modalities while awaiting their final separation.

Demobilization—Post-deployment Screening

When service members return from deployment, regardless of whether due to normal troop rotation, medical evacuation, or for administrative reasons, they receive a comprehensive screening evaluation for presence of medical and psychiatric illness. This DoD-mandated Post-Deployment Health Assessment (DD Form 2796) is performed either at the demobilization (DEMOB) site, or if a patient has been medically evacuated, at the Military Medical Center. This screening includes questions about depression, PTSD, and substance abuse. Individuals who screen positive are referred within seventy-two hours for a definitive mental health evaluation.

Service members with identified disorders are offered treatment and are evaluated for appropriate disposition. In the absence of nonpsychiatric conditions, aggressive treatment continues with the goal of retaining the individual and returning him or her to full duty. Service members are given an adequate trial of treatment before a decision is made to refer to the disability system through a MEB unless other conditions mandate referral to MEB.

Medical Evaluation Board

If a service member requires evacuation from the combat zone for combat stress symptoms, the psychiatrist must decide whether the symptoms are due to a psychiatric condition, situational problem, or personality disorder. The psychiatrist must also determine the prognosis and likelihood of response to treatment. Generally, in the absence of a personality disorder or other confounding variables, aggressive treatment of combat stress reactions is indicated. If the symptoms cannot be stabilized within a reasonable amount of time, then referral to a MEB is indicated for disability retirement.

In deciding whether and when to initiate a MEB, the treating psychiatrist must consider the military patient's length of service, previous history, current symptoms, and prognosis, as well as the time remaining on active duty for activated reservists. Junior ranking military members in their first enlistment with no prior deployment experience are likely to be referred to MEB. More seasoned military members are more likely to be monitored for up to one year with some duty limitations in an effort to retain them. Reservists who are nearing the end of their term of activation are likely to be allowed to be released from active duty (REFRAD) and referred for continued care and monitoring.

A service member may require referral to a MEB by virtue of his or her other medical conditions. When this is the case, a psychiatric addendum is performed to establish a service-connected condition, and to identify if the condition meets or does not meet medical retention standards.

One has to remain cognizant of the individual who may be attempting to manipulate the disability system in his or her favor by exaggerating symptoms, or seeking disability for conditions that are not medically unfitting. The psychiatrist must be mindful of all motivating factors and the potential for the influence of a disability-seeking culture.

Limits of Medical Authority

It is important to be aware of the limitations physicians have when treating the military patient. The military physician's role is to treat the patient, determine if the patient is medically fit to fight, and make recommendations to the patient's commander about appropriate disposition. The only area where the physician has full authority is when a condition is life-threatening, requires hospitalization, or does not meet retention standards and referral to MEB is indicated. In all other situations, the physician is a consultant to the system and can make recommendations only. Recommendations may include return to duty (RTD) without any limitations, RTD with some limitations or changes in environment, or administrative recommendations about rehabilitative or compassionate transfers, or discharge from the service.

Commanders have ultimate authority and bear ultimate responsibility for acting on recommendations. They may decide to attempt to rehabilitate a service member in his or her command despite recommendations for administrative discharge. A commander who chooses to ignore medical recommendations must review this decision with his or her higher commander. If the restrictions placed on a military member cannot be accommodated either by the nature of the mission or the individual's military occupational specialty (MOS), the commander may request a "Fitness for Duty Board" from the supporting hospital. If the service member is found fit with some limitations that constrain his or her duty performance, the commander may request evaluation by a MOS Medical Retention Board (MMRB). The MMRB can return the soldier to duty, change the soldier's MOS, or refer the soldier to the disability system.

Ethics of Military Psychiatry

Military mental health officers must struggle with the ethical issues and duties to the individual and the military. They should always be the "honest broker" in caring for military patients and making tough decisions about treatment, referral to the disability system, administrative discharges, and limitations to duty. They must balance the mission requirements with the best interest of the patient and attempt to make the recommendation that will afford the service member the best outcome and opportunity for retention. Additionally, military mental health providers have got to recognize when the demands of service cannot afford the luxury of a prolonged rehabilitative period. They are also obligated to serve the interests of the service by remaining alert to secondary gain and malingering.

Military clinicians must understand that combat is one of life's most significant traumatic events.

They have to allow some vulnerable individuals to deploy and must recognize that some will become symptomatic. Ultimately, military mental health providers are required to remain empathic to the military patient as well as the needs of the service by providing compassionate treatment for combat veterans and referring service members who cannot be rehabilitated quickly to the disability system.

Clinicians involved in the treatment of casualties returning from Operation Iraqi Freedom require an understanding of the military system in which these service members work and receive their medical care. Unlike prior conflicts, casualties from this war will likely receive treatment services in a variety of settings by providers from nonmilitary professional backgrounds.

Diversity within the military populations suggests that evacuated military patients are likely to come from different areas of the country and vary in terms of ethnic and cultural heritage. There is an increasing number of women as well. Patients' military experience may vary considerably depending upon the military component (e.g. active, reserve, or National Guard) to which these service members are assigned. They may have been exposed to a variety of different combat stressors, depending upon their site of duty, the nature of conflict to which they have been exposed, and the roles in which they have served. The literature is clear that certain psychiatric conditions, including acute stress disorders and PTSD, are not uncommon responses to individuals exposed to combat. Clinicians must be aware of other psychiatric and organic disorders that might also contribute to their presentation, however.

The military system is designed to minimize psychiatric disorders on the battlefield through pre-deployment screening and by providing mental health services in the combat setting. When evacuation is required, service members may be treated within several echelons of care that are established. Additionally, military regulation guides the appropriate evaluation of psychiatrically ill military patients. Service members with behavioral or emotional disorders may require discharge from service through the Medical Evaluation Board (MEB) process or through command-determined administrative separation.

All of these factors can contribute to the clinical condition of an evacuated soldier, airman, or sailor. An appreciation of these complex issues will serve the clinician well in evaluating and treating service members psychiatrically evacuated from theater.

TREATMENT OF THE RETURNING WAR VETERAN

Josef I. Ruzek, Ph.D., Erika Curran, M.S.W., Matthew J. Friedman, M.D., Ph.D., Fred D. Gusman, M.S.W., Steven M. Southwick, M.D., Pamela Swales, Ph.D., Robyn D. Walser, Ph.D., Patricia J. Watson, Ph.D., and Julia Whealin, Ph.D.

It is important that VA and Vet Center clinicians recognize that the skills and experience that they have developed in working with veterans with chronic PTSD will serve them well with those returning from war. Their experience in talking about trauma, educating patients and families about traumatic stress reactions, teaching skills of anxiety and anger management, facilitating mutual support among groups of veterans, and working with trauma-related guilt, will all be useful and applicable. Here, we highlight some challenges for clinicians, discuss ways in which care of these veterans may differ from our usual contexts of care, and direct attention to particular methods and materials that may be relevant to the care of the veteran recently traumatized in war.

The Helping Context: Active Duty vs. Veterans Seeking Health Care

There are a variety of differences between the contexts of care for active duty military personnel and veterans normally being served in VA that may affect the way practitioners go about their business. First, many Iraq War patients will not be seeking mental health treatment. Some will have been evacuated for mental health or medical reasons and brought to VA, perhaps reluctant to acknowledge their emotional distress and almost certainly reluctant to consider themselves as having a mental health disorder (e.g., PTSD). Second, emphasis on diagnosis as an organizing principle of mental health care is common in VA. Patients are given DSM-IV diagnoses, and diagnoses drive treatment. This approach may be contrasted with that of frontline psychiatry, in which pathologization of combat stress reactions is strenuously avoided. The strong assumption is that most will recover, and that their responses represent a severe reaction to the traumatic stress of war rather than a mental illness or disorder. According to this thinking, the "labeling" process may be counterproductive in the context of early care for Iraq War veterans. As Koshes (1996) noted, "labeling a person with an illness can reinforce the 'sick' role and delay or prevent the soldier's return to the unit or to a useful role in military or civilian life" (p. 401).

Patients themselves may have a number of incentives to minimize their distress: to hasten discharge, to accelerate a return to the family, to avoid compromising their military career or retirement. Fears about possible impact on career prospects are based in reality; indeed, some will be judged medically unfit to return to duty. Veterans may be concerned that a diagnosis of PTSD, or even acute stress disorder, in their medical record may harm their chances of future promotion, lead to a decision to not be retained, or affect type of discharge received. Some may think that the information obtained if they receive mental health treatment will be shared with their unit commanders, as is sometimes the case in the military.

To avoid legitimate concerns about possible pathologization of common traumatic stress reactions, clinicians may wish to consider avoiding, where possible, the assignment of diagnostic labels such as ASD or PTSD, and instead focus on assessing and documenting symptoms and behaviors. Diagnoses of acute or adjustment disorders may apply if symptoms warrant labeling. Concerns about confidentiality must be acknowledged and steps taken to create the conditions in which patients will feel able to talk openly about their experiences, which may include difficulties with commanders, misgivings about military operations or policies, or possible moral concerns about having participated in the war. It will be helpful for clinicians to know who will be privy to information obtained in an assessment. The role of the assessment and who will have access to what information should be discussed with concerned patients.

Active duty service members may have the option to remain on active duty or to return to the war zone. Some evidence suggests that returning to work with one's cohort group during wartime can facilitate improvement of symptoms. Although their wishes may or may not be granted, service members often have strong feelings about wanting or not wanting to return to war. For recently activated National Guard and Reservists, issues may be somewhat different (Dunning, 1996). Many in this population never planned to go to war and so may be faced with obstacles to picking up the life they "left." Whether active duty, National Guard, or Reservist, listening to and acknowledging their concerns will help empower them and inform treatment planning.

War patients entering residential mental health care will have come to the VA through a process different from that experienced by "traditional" patients. If they have been evacuated from the war zone, they will have been rapidly moved through several levels of medical triage and treatment, and treated by a variety of health care providers (Scurfield & Tice, 1991). Many will have received some mental health care in the war zone (e.g., stress debriefing) that will have been judged unsuccessful. Some veterans will perceive their need for continuing care as a sign of personal failure. Understanding their path to the VA will help the building of a relationship and the design of care.

More generally, the returning soldier is in a state of transition from war zone to home, and clinicians must seek to understand the expectations and consequences of returning home for the veteran. Is the veteran returning to an established place in society, to an economically deprived community, to a supportive spouse or cohesive military unit, to a large impersonal city, to unemployment, to financial stress, to an American public thankful for his or her sacrifice?

Whatever the circumstances, things are unlikely to be as they were:

> The deployment of the family member creates a painful void within the family system that is eventually filled (or denied) so that life can go on. . . . The family assumes that their experiences at home and the soldier's activities on the battlefield will be easily assimilated by each other at the time of reunion and that the pre-war roles will be resumed. The fact that new roles and responsibilities

may not be given up quickly upon homecoming is not anticipated. (Yerkes & Holloway, 1996, p. 31)

Learning from Vietnam Veterans with Chronic PTSD

From the perspective of work with Vietnam veterans whose lives have been greatly disrupted by their disorder, the chance to work with combat veterans soon after their war experiences represents a real opportunity to prevent the development of a disastrous life course. We have the opportunity to directly focus on traumatic stress reactions and PTSD symptom reduction (e.g., by helping veterans process their traumatic experiences, by prescribing medications) and thereby reduce the degree to which PTSD, depression, alcohol/substance misuse, or other psychological problems interfere with quality of life. We also have the opportunity to intervene directly in key areas of life functioning, to reduce the harm associated with continuing post-traumatic stress symptoms and depression if those prove resistant to treatment. The latter may possibly be accomplished via interventions focused on actively supporting family functioning in order to minimize family problems, reducing social alienation and isolation, supporting workplace functioning, and preventing use of alcohol and drugs as self-medication (a different focus than addressing chronic alcohol or drug problems).

Prevent Family Breakdown

At time of return to civilian life, they can face a variety of challenges in reentering their families, and the contrast between the fantasies and realities of homecoming (Yerkes & Holloway, 1996) can be distressing. Families themselves have been stressed and experienced problems as a result of the deployment (Norwood, Fullerton, & Hagen, 1996; Jensen & Shaw, 1996). Partners have made role adjustments while the soldier was away, and these need to be renegotiated, especially given the possible irritability and tension of the veteran (Kirkland, 1995). The possibility exists that mental health providers can reduce long-term family problems by helping veterans and their families anticipate and prepare for family challenges, involving families in treatment, providing skills training for patients (and where possible, their families) in family-relevant skills (e.g., communication, anger management, conflict resolution, parenting), providing short-term support for family members, and linking families together for mutual support.

Prevent Social Withdrawal and Isolation

PTSD also interferes with social functioning. Here the challenge is to help the veteran avoid withdrawal from others by supporting reentry into existing relationships with friends, work colleagues, and relatives, or where appropriate, assisting in development of new social relationships. The latter may be especially relevant with individuals who leave military service and transition back into civilian life. Social functioning should be routinely discussed with patients and made a target for intervention. Skills training focusing on the concrete management of specific difficult social situations may be very helpful. Also, as indicated below, clinicians should try to connect veterans with other veterans in order to facilitate the development of social networks.

Prevent Problems with Employment

Associated with chronic combat-related PTSD have been high rates of job turnover and general difficulty in maintaining employment, often attributed by veterans themselves to anger and irritability, difficulties with authority, PTSD symptoms, and substance abuse. Steady employment, however, is likely to be one predictor of better long-term functioning, as it can reduce financial stresses, provide a source of meaningful activity and self-esteem, and give opportunities for companionship and friendship. In some cases, clinicians can provide valuable help by supporting the military or civilian work functioning of veterans, by teaching skills of maintaining or, in the case of those leaving the military, finding of employment, or facilitating job-related support groups.

Prevent Alcohol and Drug Abuse

The comorbidity of PTSD with alcohol and drug problems in veterans is well established (Ruzek, 2003). Substance abuse adds to the problems caused by PTSD and interferes with key roles and relationships, impairs coping, and impairs entry into and ongoing participation in treatment. PTSD providers are aware of the need to routinely screen and assess for alcohol and drug use, and are knowledgeable about alcohol and drug (especially 12 Step) treatment. Many are learning, as well, about the potential usefulness of integrated PTSD-substance abuse treatment, and the availability of manualized treatments for this dual disorder. Seeking Safety, a structured group protocol for trauma-relevant coping skills training (Najavits, 2002), is seeing increased use in VA and should be considered as a treatment option for Iraq War veterans who have substance use disorders along with problematic traumatic stress responses. In addition, for many newly returning Iraq War veterans, it will be important to supplement traditional abstinence-oriented treatments with attention to milder alcohol problems, and in particular to initiate preventive interventions to reduce drinking or prevent acceleration of alcohol consumption as a response to PTSD symptoms (Bien, Miller, & Tonigan, 1993). For *all* returning veterans, it will be useful to provide education about safe drinking practices and the relationship between traumatic stress reactions and substance abuse.

General Considerations in Care

Connect with the Returning Veteran

As with all mental health counseling, the relationship between veteran and helper will be the starting point for care. Forming a working alliance with some returnees may be challenging, however, because most newly returned veterans may be, as Litz notes, "defended, formal, respectful, laconic, and cautious" and reluctant to work with the mental health professional. Especially in the context of recent exposure to war, validation (Kirkland, 1995) of the veteran's experiences and concerns will be crucial. Discussion of "war zone," not "combat," stress may be warranted because some traumatic stressors (e.g., body handling, sexual assault) may not involve war fighting as such. Thought needs to be given to making the male-centric hospital system hospitable for women, especially for women who have experienced sexual assault in the war zone, for whom simply walking onto the grounds of a VA hospital with the ubiquitous presence of men may create feelings of vulnerability and anxiety.

Practitioners should work from a patient-centered perspective, and take care to find out the current concerns of the patient (e.g., fear of returning to the war zone, concerns about having been evacuated and what this means, worries about reactions of unit, fear of career ramifications, concern about reactions of family, concerns about returning to active duty). One advantage of such an orientation is that it will assist with the development of a helping relationship.

Connect Veterans with Each Other

In treatment of chronic PTSD, veterans often report that perhaps their most valued experience was the opportunity to connect in friendship and support with other vets. This is unlikely to be different for returning Iraq War veterans, who may benefit greatly from connection both with each other and with veterans of other conflicts. Fortunately, this is a strength of VA and Vet Center clinicians, who routinely and skillfully bring veterans together.

Offer Practical Help with Specific Problems

Returning veterans are likely to feel overwhelmed with problems related to workplace, family and friends, finances, physical health, and so on.

These problems will be drawing much of their attention away from the tasks of therapy, and may create a climate of continuing stress that interferes with resolution of symptoms. The presence of continuing negative consequences of war deployment may help maintain post-traumatic stress reactions. Rather than treating these issues as distractions from the task at hand, clinicians can provide a valuable service by helping veterans identify, prioritize, and execute action steps to address their specific problems.

Attend to Broad Needs of the Person

Wolfe, Keane, and Young (1996) put forward several suggestions for clinicians serving Persian Gulf War veterans that are also important in the context of the Iraq War. They recommended attention to the broad range of traumatic experience. They similarly recommended broad clinical attention to the impact of both pre-military and post-military stressors on adjustment. For example, history of trauma places those exposed to trauma in the war zone at risk for development of PTSD, and in some cases war experiences will activate emotions experienced during earlier events. Finally, recognition and referral for assessment of the broad range of physical health concerns and complaints that may be reported by returning veterans is important. Mental health providers must remember that increased health symptom reporting is unlikely to be exclusively psychogenic in origin (Proctor et al., 1998).

Methods of Care: Overview

Management of acute stress reactions and problems faced by recently returned veterans are highlighted below. Methods of care for the Iraq War veteran with PTSD will be similar to those provided to veterans with chronic PTSD.

Education about Post-traumatic Stress Reactions

Education is a key component of care for the veteran returning from war experience and is intended to improve understanding and recognition of symptoms, reduce fear and shame about symptoms, and, generally, "normalize" his or her experience. It should also provide the veteran with a clear understanding of how recovery is thought to take place, what will happen in treatment, and, as appropriate, the role of medication.

With such understanding, stress reactions may seem more predictable and fears about long-term effects can be reduced. Education in the context of relatively recent traumatization (weeks or months) should include the conception that many symptoms are the result of psychobiological reactions to extreme stress and that, with time, these reactions, in most cases, will diminish.

Reactions should be interpreted as responses to overwhelming stress rather than as personal weakness or inadequacy. In fact, some recent research (e.g., Steil & Ehlers, 2000) suggests that survivors' own responses to their stress symptoms will in part determine the degree of distress associated with those symptoms and whether they will remit. Whether, for example, post-trauma intrusions cause distress may depend in part on their meaning for the person (e.g., "I'm going crazy").

Training in Coping Skills

Returning veterans experiencing recurrent intrusive thoughts and images, anxiety and panic in response to trauma cues, and feelings of guilt or intense anger are likely to feel relatively powerless to control their emotions and thoughts. This helpless feeling is in itself a trauma reminder. Because loss of control is so central to trauma and its attendant emotions, interventions that restore self-efficacy are especially useful.

Coping skills training is a core element in the repertoire of many VA and Vet Center mental health providers. Some skills that may be effective in treating Iraq War veterans include anxiety management (breathing retraining and relaxation), emotional "grounding," anger management, and communication. However, the days, weeks, and months following the return home may pose specific situational challenges; therefore, a careful assessment of the veteran's current experience must guide selection of skills. For example, training in communication skills might focus on the problem experienced by a veteran in expressing positive feelings toward a partner (often associated with emotional numbing); anger management could help the veteran better respond to others in the immediate environment who do not support the war.

Whereas education helps survivors understand their experience and know what to do about it, coping skills training should focus on helping them know *how* to do the things that will support recovery. It relies on a cycle of instruction that includes education, demonstration, rehearsal with feedback and coaching, and repeated practice. It includes regular between-session task assignments with diary self-monitoring and real-world practice of skills. It is this repeated practice and real-world experience that begins to empower the veteran to better manage his or her challenges (see Najavits, 2002, for a useful manual of trauma-related coping skills).

Exposure Therapy

Exposure therapy is among the best-supported treatments for PTSD (Foa et al., 2000). It is designed to help veterans effectively confront their trauma-related emotions and painful memories, and can be distinguished from simple discussion of traumatic experience in that it emphasizes *repeated* verbalization of traumatic memories (see Foa & Rothbaum, 1998, for a detailed exposition of the treatment). Patients are exposed to their own individualized fear stimuli repetitively, until fear responses are consistently diminished. Often, in-session exposure is supplemented by therapist-assigned and monitored self-exposure to the memories or situations associated with traumatization. In most treatment settings, exposure is delivered as part of a more comprehensive "package" treatment; it is usually combined with traumatic stress education, coping skills training, and, especially, cognitive restructuring (see below). Exposure therapy can help correct faulty perceptions of danger, improve perceived self-control of memories and accompanying negative emotions, and strengthen adaptive coping responses under conditions of distress.

Cognitive Restructuring

Cognitive therapy or restructuring, one of the best-validated PTSD treatments (Foa et al., 2000), is designed to help the patient review and challenge distressing trauma-related beliefs. It focuses on educating participants about the relationships between thoughts and emotions, exploring common negative thoughts held by trauma survivors, identifying personal negative beliefs, developing alternative interpretations or judgments, and practicing new thinking. This is a systematic approach that goes well beyond simple discussion of beliefs to include individual assessment, self-monitoring of thoughts, homework assignments, and real-world practice. In particular, it may be a most helpful approach to a range of emotions other than fear—guilt, shame, anger, depression—that may trouble veterans. For example, anger may be fueled by negative beliefs (e.g., about perceived lack of preparation or training for war experiences, about harm done to their civilian career, about perceived lack of support from civilians). Cognitive therapy may also be helpful in helping veterans cope with distressing changed perceptions of personal identity that may be associated with participation in war or loss of wartime identity upon return (Yerkes & Holloway, 1996).

A useful resource is the *Cognitive Processing Therapy* manual developed by Resick and Schnicke (1993), which incorporates extensive cognitive restructuring and limited exposure. Although designed for application to rape-related PTSD, the methods can be easily adapted for use with veterans. Kubany's (1998) work on trauma-related guilt may be helpful in addressing veterans' concerns about harming or causing death to civilians.

Family Counseling

Mental health professionals within VA and Vet Centers have a long tradition of working with family members of veterans with PTSD. This same work, including family education, weekend family workshops, couples counseling, family therapy, parenting classes, or training in conflict resolution, will be very important with Iraq War veterans.

Pharmacotherapy

Pharmacologic Treatment of Acute Stress Reactions

Pharmacological treatment for acute stress reactions (within one month of the trauma) is generally reserved for individuals who remain symptomatic after having already received brief crisis-oriented psychotherapy. This approach is in line with the deliberate attempt by military professionals to avoid medicalizing stress-related symptoms and to adhere to a strategy of immediacy, proximity, and positive expectancy.

Prior to receiving medication for stress-related symptoms, the war zone survivor should have a thorough psychiatric and medical examination, with special emphasis on medical disorders that can manifest with psychiatric symptoms (e.g., subdural hematoma, hyperthyroidism), potential psychiatric disorders (e.g., acute stress disorder, depression, psychotic disorders, panic disorder), use of alcohol and substances of abuse, use of prescribed and over-the-counter medication, and possible drug allergies. It is important to assess the full range of potential psychiatric disorders, and not just PTSD, since many symptomatic service personnel will be at an age when first episodes of schizophrenia, mania, depression, and panic disorder are often seen.

In some cases a clinician may need to prescribe psychotropic medications even before completing the medical or psychiatric examination. The acute use of medications may be necessary when the patient is dangerous, extremely agitated, or psychotic. In such circumstances the patient should be taken to an emergency room; short-acting benzodiazepines (e.g., lorazepam) or high-potency neuroleptics (e.g., Haldol) with minimal sedative, anticholinergic, and orthostatic side effects may prove effective. Atypical neuroleptics (e.g., risperidone) may also be useful for treating aggression.

When a decision has been made to use medication for acute stress reactions, rational choices may include benzodiazepines, antiadrenergics, or antidepressants. Shortly after traumatic exposure, the brief prescription of benzodiazepines (four days or less) has been shown to reduce extreme arousal and anxiety and to improve sleep. However, early and prolonged use of benzodiazepines is contraindicated, since benzodiazepine use for two weeks or longer has actually has been associated with a higher rate of subsequent PTSD.

Although antiadrenergic agents including clonidine, guanfacine, prazosin, and propranolol have been recommended (primarily through open nonplacebo controlled treatment trials) for the treatment of hyperarousal, irritable aggression, intrusive memories, nightmares, and insomnia in survivors with chronic PTSD, there is only suggestive preliminary evidence of their efficacy as an acute treatment. Of importance, antiadrenergic agents should be prescribed judiciously for trauma survivors with cardiovascular disease due to potential hypotensive effects and these agents should also be tapered, rather than discontinued abruptly, in order to avoid rebound hypertension.

Further, because antiadrenergic agents might interfere with counterregulatory hormone responses to hypoglycemia, they should not be prescribed to survivors with diabetes.

Finally, the use of antidepressants may make sense within four weeks of war, particularly when trauma-related depressive symptoms are prominent and debilitating. To date, there has been one published report on the use of antidepressants for the treatment of acute stress disorder. Recently trauma-tized children meeting criteria for acute stress disorder, who were treated with imipramine for two weeks, experienced significantly greater symptom reduction than children who were prescribed chloral hydrate.

Pharmacologic Treatment of Post-traumatic Stress Disorder

Pharmacotherapy is rarely used as a stand-alone treatment for PTSD and is usually combined with psychological treatment. The following text briefly presents recommendations for the pharmacotherapeutic treatment of PTSD. Findings from subsequent large-scale trials with paroxetine have demon-strated that SSRI treatment is clearly effective both for men in general and for combat veterans suffering with PTSD.

We recommend SSRIs as first-line medications for PTSD pharmacother-apy in men and women with military-related PTSD. SSRIs appear to be effec-tive for all three PTSD symptom clusters in both men and women who have experienced a variety of severe traumas and they are also effective in treating a variety of comorbid psychiatric disorders, such as major depression and panic disorder, which are commonly seen in individuals suffering with PTSD. Additionally, the side effect profile with SSRIs is relatively benign (compared to most psychotropic medications) although arousal and insom-nia may be experienced early on for some patients with PTSD.

Second-line medications include nefazadone, tricyclic antidepressants (TCAs), and monoamine oxidase inhibitors (MAOIs). Evidence favoring the use of these agents is not as compelling as for SSRIs because many fewer subjects have been tested at this point. The best evidence from open trials supports the use of nefazadone, which, like SSRIs, promotes serotonergic ac-tions and is less likely than SSRIs to cause insomnia or sexual dysfunction. Trazadone, which has limited efficacy as a stand-alone treatment, has proven very useful as augmentation therapy with SSRIs; its sedating properties make it a useful bedtime medication that can antagonize SSRI-induced insomnia. Despite some favorable evidence of the efficacy of monoamine oxidase inhib-itors (MAOIs), these compounds have received little experimental attention since 1990.

Venlafaxine and bupropion cannot be recommended because they have not been tested systematically in clinical trials.

There is a strong rationale from laboratory research to consider antiadren-ergic agents. It is hoped that more extensive testing will establish their useful-ness for PTSD patients. The best research on this class of agents has focused on prazosin, which has produced marked reduction in traumatic nightmares, improved sleep, and global improvement in veterans with PTSD. Hypotension and sedation need to be monitored. Patients should not be abruptly discontinued from antiadrenergics. Despite suggestive theoretical considerations and clinical findings, there is only a small amount of evidence to support the use of carbamazepine or valproate with PTSD patients. Further, the complexities of clinical management with these effective anticonvulsants have shifted current attention to newer agents (e.g., gabapentin, lamotrigine, and topirimate), which have yet to be tested systematically with PTSD patients.

Benzodiazepines cannot be recommended for patients with PTSD. They do not appear to have efficacy against core PTSD symptoms. No studies have demonstrated efficacy for PTSD-specific symptoms.

Conventional antipsychotics cannot be recommended for PTSD patients. Preliminary results suggest, however, that atypical antipsychotics may be useful, especially to augment treatment with first- or second-line medications, especially for patients with intense hypervigilance or paranoia, agitation, dissociation, or brief psychotic reactions associated with their PTSD. As for side effects, all atypicals may produce weight gain, and olanzapine treatment has been linked to the onset of Type II diabetes mellitus.

General Guidelines

Pharmacotherapy should be initiated with SSRI agents. Patients who cannot tolerate SSRIs or who show no improvement might benefit from nefazadone, MAOIs, or TCAs.

For patients who exhibit a partial response to SSRIs, one should consider continuation or augmentation. A recent trial with sertraline showed that approximately half of all patients who failed to exhibit a successful clinical response after twelve weeks of sertraline treatment, did respond when SSRI treatment was extended for another twenty-four weeks. Practically speaking, clinicians and patients usually will be reluctant to stick with an ineffective medication for thirty-six weeks, as in this experiment. Therefore, augmentation strategies seem to make sense. Here are a few suggestions based on clinical experience and pharmacological "guesstimates," rather than on hard evidence:

- Excessively aroused, hyperreactive, or dissociating patients might be helped by augmentation with an antiadrenergic agent.

- Labile, impulsive, and/or aggressive patients might benefit from augmentation with an anticonvulsant.
- Fearful, hypervigilant, paranoid, and psychotic patients might benefit from an atypical antipsychotic.

Integrating into Existing Specialized PTSD Services

War service members with stress-related problems may need to be integrated into existing VA PTSD Residential Rehabilitation Programs or other VA mental health programs. Approaches to this integration of psychiatric evacuees will vary and each receiving site will need to determine its own "best fit" model for provision of services and integration of veterans. At the National Center's PTSD Residential Rehabilitation Program in the VA Palo Alto Health Care System, it is anticipated that Iraq War patients will generally be integrated with the rest of the milieu (e.g., for community meetings, affect management classes, conflict resolution, communication skills training), with the exception of identified treatment components. The latter elements of treatment, in which Iraq War veterans will work together, will include process, case management, and acute stress/PTSD education groups (and, if delivered in groups, exposure therapy, cognitive restructuring, and family/couples counseling). The thoughtful mixing of returning veterans with veterans from other wars/conflicts is likely, in general, to enhance the treatment experience of both groups.

Practitioner Issues

Working with Iraq War veterans affected by war zone trauma is likely to be emotionally difficult for therapists. It is likely to bring up many feelings and concerns—reactions to stories of death and great suffering, judgments about the morality of the war, reactions to patients who have killed, feelings of personal vulnerability, feelings of therapeutic inadequacy, perceptions of a lack of preparation for acute care—that may affect ability to listen empathically to the patient and maintain the therapeutic relationship (Sonnenberg, 1996). Koshes (1996) suggested that those at greatest risk for strong personal reactions might be young, inexperienced staff who are close in age to patients and more likely to identify with them, and technicians or paraprofessional workers who may have less formal education about the challenges associated with treating these patients but who actually spend the most time with patients. Regardless of degree of experience, all mental health workers must monitor themselves and practice active self-care, and managers must ensure that training, support, and supervision are part of the environment in which care is offered.

* * *

Treatment of Medical Casualty Evacuees

Josef I. Ruzek, Ph.D. and Harold Kudler, M.D.

Men and women evacuated from the war zone due to physical injury are at higher risk than other service personnel for development of PTSD and other trauma-related problems. If the VA serves as a care facility for Iraq War medical casualties, it will be important that clinical attention be given not just to their physical recovery and health, but to their mental health needs. Failure to do so may be to lose a significant and unique opportunity for early intervention to prevent development of more chronic emotional and behavioral problems. In this section we outline some considerations related to the integration of mental health care with physical care of recently evacuated Iraq War veterans.

This kind of activity represents a challenge for VA mental health professionals. While VA PTSD, behavioral medicine, and other mental health practitioners are familiar with delivery of traumatic stress assessment and treatment to help-seeking veterans with chronic PTSD or general health problems, they are less likely to have delivered such services to individuals who have been injured during very recent exposure to traumas of war. More generally, focus on treatment of physical problems is often accompanied by a strong desire on the part of both patient and provider to avoid discussing emotional issues (Scurfield & Tice, 1991).

Offering Comprehensive Care

Traumatic stress–related interventions should be presented as part of *routine* care given to all patients, and framed as a component of a comprehensive response to the needs of the veteran, in which the whole person is treated. Stress-related education will be helpful for all patients, including those not showing traumatic stress reactions, because health problems inevitably bring stress and challenges in coping.

Most medical casualties will not be seeking mental health care. Many can be expected to be reluctant to acknowledge their emotional distress and some will be concerned that a mental health diagnosis (e.g., PTSD) in their medical record may harm their chances of future promotion.

Therefore, clinicians need to minimize mental health jargon, avoid pathologizing common stress reactions, and be thoughtful about assignment of DSM-IV diagnoses.

Helping Services

In civilian work with patients receiving hospital care for traumatic injury, mental health services are not routinely delivered. However, the VA service delivery context has a number of potential advantages compared with other post-trauma intervention settings (e.g., disaster mental health services, hospital trauma centers). These advantages are based on the availability of experienced mental health professionals with expertise in traumatic stress care, and include opportunities for routine screening, routine patient education, careful individual assessment, psychiatric consultation, individualized mental health treatment with multisession contact, family involvement in care, and mobilization of group support from other hospitalized Iraq War veterans and veterans of other wars. In other words, there is the opportunity to deliver a level of intensity of care that is matched to the veteran, rather than relying on a one-size-fits-all, brief intervention.

Routine Screening

Proactive care of returning veterans will require that they be routinely screened for post-traumatic distress and mental health problems. In the absence of direct enquiry about distress and symptoms, it is likely that many individuals with significant problems will be missed.

Iraq War veterans, like other populations, cannot be expected to spontaneously disclose their distressing war experiences and associated problems. Several paper-and-pencil screens are available. It is important for mental health professionals to become a routine presence on medical and surgical settings. Rather than appear with a series of medical questions, it is more helpful to present as a member of the team who would like to be helpful and who has time to listen, answer questions, or help with a problem.

This approach, sometimes referred to as "therapy by walking around," is consistent with the importance of not pathologizing reactions to overwhelming stress. It fosters trust and openness and still offers opportunities, if needed, for further assessment, triage, and treatment.

Routine Patient Education

A good way to present services is to frame them as patient education in stress management. Patient education will offer a primary means of initiating proactive mental health care. Patients may differ greatly in their receptiveness to such discussions, and staff must remain sensitive to the state of readiness of each individual patient, and vary their approach and degree of discussion accordingly. However, it is important to initiate some discussion; failure to do so may encourage emotional avoidance and miss a significant and perhaps unique opportunity to offer preventive care. Group education "classes" can be helpful in making such discussions more acceptable to patients. They also provide opportunities for more receptive patients to model open communication and disclosure of personal stress reactions, thoughts, and feelings.

Assessment

Administration of screening tools and patient education activities offer chances to determine which veterans will benefit from a more detailed assessment. In assessing stressors experienced in the war zone, clinicians should also take care to actively inquire about experiences associated with medical care and evacuation. Those being evacuated are often exposed to the suffering and death of other wounded vets. Preliminary work in the civilian sector suggests that the majority of injured patients value the opportunity to undergo a comprehensive psychosocial assessment during hospitalization, despite any inconvenience or distress caused by the process (Ruzek & Zatzick, 2000).

Psychiatric Consultation

In addition to their role in providing the various helping services listed in this section, consultation with psychiatry is especially important given the wide range of possible patient presentations and possible usefulness of psychotropic medications. In addition to ASD/PTSD, depression, and substance abuse, a large variety of mental health disorders (including other anxiety disorders, adjustment disorders, somatoform disorders, psychosomatic disorders, conversion disorders, dissociative amnesia disorder, and dissociative identity disorder) may be associated with exposure to combat and other war zone stressors. Medications may be useful in treating traumatic stress symptoms, associated disorders, and associated problems (e.g., sleep, nightmares). Mental health staff need to partner with Med/Surg nursing staff because these are the people who will know which patients are sleeping well, crying out in their dreams, having problems before or after family meetings, and so on. Chaplain service is another valuable partner as they are a regular presence on Med/Surg units and because military personnel are used to sharing stress-related issues with military chaplains. It is essential to promote a team approach in which mental health can be a full partner in the response to medical and/or surgical patients.

Individualized Treatment

If treatments involving exploration of traumatic experiences, cognitive restructuring, or skills training are delivered, they should include multiple treatment sessions. Where patients report symptoms consistent with a diagnosis of acute stress disorder or PTSD, cognitive-behavioral treatments, comprised of education, breathing training/relaxation, imaginal and *in vivo* exposure, and cognitive restructuring, should be considered, given the evidence for their effectiveness with other trauma populations with ASD (Bryant, Harvey, Dang, Sackville, & Basten, 1998; Bryant, Sackville, Dang, Moulds, & Guthrie, 1999) and PTSD (e.g., Rothbaum, Meadows, Resick, & Foy, 2000). Existing alcohol and drug problems should be treated, and brief preventive alcohol interventions should be routinely administered to all other veterans who consume alcohol, given the strong association between PTSD and alcohol problems (Ouimette & Brown, 2002). In the civilian sector, a brief alcohol intervention provided to heavy-drinking hospital trauma center patients resulted in significant decreases in drinking levels (Gentilello et al., 1999).

In addition to such treatment, mental health practitioners can help injured and ill returnees cope more effectively with some of the specific challenges associated with their medical condition.

They can help patients prepare for medical procedures (e.g., surgery) that are often experienced as trauma reminders. Such help may be especially important with sexual assault survivors, because health care examinations may present powerful triggers for traumatic stress reactions. For example, Resnick, Acierno, Holmes, Kilpatrick, and Jager (1999) developed a seventeen-minute educational videotape to prepare sexually assaulted women to undergo forensic rape examinations. Shown to women immediately before the exam, the video provided information about exam procedures, showed model victims calmly completing the procedures, and instructed viewers in self-directed exposure exercises, ways of reducing avoidance, and ways of improving mood and lowering anxiety. Women viewing the video had significantly lower postexam distress ratings and anxiety symptoms than nonviewers. Mental health professionals can also teach ways of managing pain, an important goal given that post-trauma pain has sometimes been found to predict PTSD.

Generally, illness and the patient role are often associated with perceptions of lack of control, and providers need to find ways to involve their patients as active participants in their medical care, by giving information about medical conditions and procedures and maximizing patient choice wherever possible.

Family Involvement in Care

One of the primary concerns and tasks facing the veteran is reconnection with the family. This may present some challenges for those evacuated due to injury or illness. Veterans and family members alike may feel awkward and unsure of how to talk to each other about what has happened. Scurfield and Tice (1991) identified a variety of family concerns and difficulties, including that families may feel embarrassment or shame about the emotional "breakdown" of the veteran, anger at the veteran for abandoning the family or jeopardizing its financial security, or guilt about having encouraged or allowed the veteran to go to war. Some hospitalized patients may not wish to have immediate contact with their families. Whatever the situation, mental health professionals can provide a valuable service in helping prepare patients and families alike for their initial reunion, and helping them address their emerging challenges.

Group Support

Groups are likely to be helpful for and well received by Iraq War veterans. They may create a forum in which stress reactions can be normalized, education delivered, support given and received, and skills practiced. Groups can be expected to foster a sense of belonging to counter the feelings of loneliness and isolation so often experienced by returning veterans (Wain & Jaccard, 1996). Providers may wish to consider integrating Iraq War service personnel into existing specialized PTSD group services, to help the younger veterans connect with veterans of other conflicts, and to provide them with a valuable perspective on their problems.

Support for Health Care Providers

In addition to consulting with the medical care team and providing direct education, assessment, treatment, and group therapy services, mental health workers can offer a valuable service in training and providing structured emotional support for health care workers serving casualties. Experience in military medical programs and in postdisaster situations such as the aftermath of the attacks of September 11 clearly points to the importance of taking good care of your staff. This is primarily accomplished by making sure that they take good care of themselves. Extended tours of duty are common in emergency situations but individual staff can only function under such conditions for so long. It is important to cultivate a professional culture in which people take regular breaks, get reasonable sleep and food, and have regular contact with their own colleagues, friends, and family in order to support their continued work with casualties and their families.

*   *   *

PTSD IN WAR VETERANS: IMPLICATIONS FOR PRIMARY CARE

Annabel Prins, Ph.D., Rachel Kimerling, Ph.D., and Gregory Leskin, Ph.D.

During and after the Iraq War, primary care providers may notice changes in their patient population. There may be an increased number of veterans or active duty military personnel returning from the war. There also may be increased contact with family members of active duty personnel, including family members who have lost a loved one in the war or family members of individuals missing in action or taken prisoner of war. In addition, there may be increased distress in veterans of other wars, conflicts, and peacekeeping missions.

All of these patients may be experiencing symptoms of post-traumatic stress disorder (PTSD):

- Veterans and active duty military personnel may have witnessed or participated in frightening and upsetting aspects of combat.
- Veterans and active duty military personnel may have experienced military-related sexual trauma during their service.
- Family members may suffer traumatic stress by hearing about frightening

or upsetting events that happened to loved ones, or from the loss or fears of loss related to family members missing or deceased.

- Other veterans may be reminded of frightening and upsetting experiences from past wars, which can exacerbate traumatic stress responses.

These types of stress reactions often lead people to increase their medical utilization. Because far fewer people experiencing traumatic stress reactions seek mental health services, primary care providers are the health professionals with whom individuals with PTSD are most likely to come into contact.

What Do Primary Care Practitioners Need to Know about PTSD?

Patients Want Primary Care Providers to Acknowledge Their Traumatic Experiences and Responses

- Over 90 percent of patients indicate that traumatic experiences and responses are important and relevant to their primary care.
- Over 90 percent of patients in VA primary care settings will have experienced at least one traumatic event in their life. Most will have experienced four or more.
- The relationship between trauma exposure and increased health care utilization appears to be mediated by the diagnosis of PTSD.
- Thus, primary care practitioners should be aware of the essential features of PTSD: reexperiencing symptoms (e.g., nightmares, intrusive thoughts), avoidance of trauma cues, numbing/detachment from others, and hyperarousal (e.g., increased startle, hypervigilance).

PTSD Can Be Detected in Primary Care Settings

- The Primary Care PTSD (PC-PTSD) screen can be used to detect PTSD in primary care.
- Endorsement of any three items is associated with a diagnostic accuracy of .85 (sensitivity .78; specificity .87) and indicates the need for additional assessment.

PTSD Can Be Effectively Managed in Primary Care Settings

By recognizing patients with PTSD and other trauma-related symptoms you can

- Provide patients and their family members with educational materials that help them understand that their feelings are connected to the Iraq War and its consequences.
- Validate patients' distress, and help them know that their feelings are not unusual in these circumstances.
- When appropriate, initiate treatment for PTSD or mental health consultation.

What Can Primary Care Providers Do for Their Patients?

Determine the Patient's Status in Relationship to the War

By assessing the patient's status in relation to the war, primary care providers acknowledge the relevance and importance of this event. Example questions include

> "Have you recently returned from the Persian Gulf? How has your adjustment been?"
> "Do you have family members or friends who are currently in the Persian Gulf? How are you dealing with their absence?"
> "How has the war in Iraq affected your functioning?"

Acknowledge the Patient's Struggles

Regardless of their specific relationship to the war, primary care providers should recognize and normalize distress associated with war. Example statements include

> "I am so sorry that you are struggling with this."
> "I can appreciate how difficult this is for you."
> "You are not the only patient I have who is struggling with this."
> "It's not easy, is it?"

Assess for PTSD Symptoms

The PC-PTSD can be used either as a self-report measure or through interview. It can be a standard part of a patient information form or introduced as follows:

> "I would like to know if you are experiencing any specific symptoms."
> "It is not uncommon for people to have certain types of reactions. I would like to know if . . ."

Be Aware of How Trauma May Impact on Medical Care

The specific health problems associated with PTSD are varied and suggest multiple etiologies; neurobiological, psychological, and behavioral factors are likely explanations. Research has increasingly demonstrated that PTSD can lead to neurobiological dysregulation, altering the functioning of catecholamine, hypothalamic-pituitary-adrenocorticoid, endogenous opioid, thyroid, immune, and neurotransmitter systems.

Exposure to traumatic stress is associated with increased health complaints, health service utilization, morbidity, and mortality.

PTSD appears to be a key mechanism that accounts for the association between trauma and poor health.

PTSD and exposure to traumatic experiences are associated with a variety of health-threatening behaviors, such as alcohol and drug use, risky sexual practices, and suicidal ideation and gestures.

PTSD is associated with an increased number of both lifetime and current physical symptoms, and PTSD severity is positively related to self-reports of physical conditions.

Determine If and How Trauma Responses Can Be Managed in PC

The delivery of mental health care is possible in the general or primary care setting. According to this approach, brief psychotherapeutic, psychoeducational, and pharmacological services are delivered as a "first line" intervention to primary care patients. If a patient fails to respond to this level of intervention, or obviously needs specialized treatment (e.g., presence of psychotic symptoms or severe dissociative symptoms), the patient is referred to mental health emergency, outpatient mental health intake coordinator, or PTSD program.

Procedures to Follow If Patient Demonstrates PTSD Symptoms during Medical Examination

Medical examinations or procedures may cause the patient to feel anxious or panicky. The following techniques may help in addressing trauma-related symptoms that arise in the medical setting:

- Speak in a calm, matter-of-fact voice.
- Reassure the patient that everything is okay.

- Remind the patient that he or she is in a safe place and his or her care and well-being are a top priority.
- Explain medical procedures and check with the patient (e.g., "Are you ok?").
- Ask (or remind) the patient where he or she is right now.
- If the patient is experiencing flashbacks, remind him or her that they are in a doctor's office at a specific time in a specific place (grounding).
- Offer the patient a drink of water, an extra gown, or a warm or cold wash cloth for the face, anything that will make the patient feel more like his or her usual self.
- Any assistance and sensitivity on the part of the primary care provider can help reinforce an effective and positive alliance with the patient.

Additional Resources

To learn more about screening and treatment for PTSD in primary care settings, additional educational materials are available at the following websites:

Post-Traumatic Stress Disorder: Implications for Primary Care Independent Study Course, Veterans Health Initiative: vaww.sites.lrn.va.gov/vhi (available through VA intranet only).

National Center for PTSD website: www.ptsd.va.gov/professional/index.asp.

National Institute for Mental Health information on PTSD: www.nimh.nih.gov/health/topics/post-traumatic-stress-disorder-ptsd/index.shtml.

6

Barriers to Seeking Care

CONFRONT MENTAL HEALTH STIGMA

Mental health problems are not a sign of weakness. The reality is that injuries, including psychological injuries, affect the strong and the brave just like everyone else. Some of the most successful officers and enlisted personnel have experienced these problems.

But stigma about mental health issues can be a huge barrier for people who need help. Finding the solution to your problem is a sign of strength and maturity. Getting assistance from others is sometimes the only way to solve something. For example, if you cannot scale a wall on your own and need a comrade to do so, you use them! Knowing when and how to get help is actually part of military training.

PTSD is not the only serious problem that can occur after deployment. Watch out for signs of these other conditions in yourself and your comrades.

DEPRESSION

We all experience sadness or feel down from time to time. That's a normal part of being human. Depression, however, is different. It lasts longer and is more serious than normal sadness or grief. Common symptoms include

- Feeling down or sad more days than not
- Losing interest in hobbies or activities that you used to find enjoyable or fun
- Being excessively low in energy and/or overly tired
- Feeling that things are never going to get better

DEPRESSION
A NATIONAL CENTER FOR PTSD FACT SHEET
   Jennifer Gregg, Ph.D.

Depression is a common problem in which severe and long-lasting feelings of sadness or other problems get in the way of a person's ability to function. In any given year, as many as 18.8 million American adults—9.5 percent of the adult population—experience some type of depression.

Unlike a blue mood that comes and goes, depression is a persistent problem that affects the way a person eats and sleeps, thinks about things, and feels about him- or herself.

What Are the Symptoms of Depression?

The symptoms of depression can vary quite a bit, but most people who experience depression feel down or sad more days than not, or find that things in their life no longer seem enjoyable or interesting. Additionally, people with depression may notice changes in their sleeping, eating, concentration, or feelings about themselves, and may find themselves feeling hopeless. These symptoms typically last for at least two weeks without letting up.

What Causes Depression?

Depression has many causes. Difficulty coping with painful experiences or losses contributes to depression. People returning from a war zone often experience painful memories, feelings of guilt or regret about their war experiences, or have a tough time readjusting back to normal life.

Trouble coping with these feelings and experiences can lead to depression. Some types of depression run in families, and depression is often associated with chemical imbalances and other changes in the brain.

How Is Depression Treated?

There are many treatment options for depression. An evaluation should be done by a health care professional to help determine which type of treatment is best for an individual. Typically, milder forms of depression are treated by psychotherapy, and more severe depression is treated with medications or a combination of psychotherapy and medication. Your doctor can help you determine which treatment is best for you.

Psychotherapy

There are a number of types of psychotherapy (or talk therapy) that are used to treat depression. These treatments may involve just a few sessions, or may last ten to twenty weeks or longer. Psychotherapy treatments tend to focus on helping patients learn about their problems and resolve them, through working with a therapist and learning new patterns of behavior to help decrease depression. Two of the main types of psychotherapy for depression are interpersonal therapy and cognitive-behavioral therapy. Interpersonal therapy focuses on the patient's relationships with other people, and how these relationships may cause and maintain depression. Cognitive-behavioral treatments help patients change negative styles of thinking and acting that can lead to depression.

Medication

In addition to psychotherapy, there are several types of antidepressant medications used to treat depression. These include selective serotonin reuptake inhibitors (SSRIs), tricyclics, and monoamine oxidase inhibitors (MAOIs). The newer medications for treating depression, such as the SSRIs, generally have fewer side effects than older types of medications. A health care provider may try more than one type of medication, or may increase the dosage, to find a treatment that works. Improvements in symptoms of depression typically occur after the medication is taken regularly for three to four weeks, although in some medications it may take as long as eight weeks for the full effect to occur.

Antidepressant medications are typically safe and effective. They help patients feel less depressed and generally do not make people feel "drugged" or different during their daily lives. The side effects of depression medications vary depending on the medication, and can include dry mouth, constipation, bladder problems, sexual problems, blurred vision, dizziness, drowsiness, headache, nausea, nervousness, or insomnia. Because of side effects or because they begin feeling better, patients are often tempted to stop taking their medication too soon. Some medications must be stopped slowly to give your body time to readjust to not having the medication. Never stop taking an antidepressant without consulting your doctor.

What Can I Do about Feelings of Depression?

Depression can make a person feel exhausted, worthless, helpless, hopeless, and sad. These feelings can make you feel as though you are never going to feel better, or that you should just give up. It is important to realize that these negative thoughts and feelings are part of depression, and often fade as treatment begins working. In the meantime, here is a list of things to try to improve your mood:

- Talk with your doctor or health care provider.
- Talk with family and friends, and let them help you.
- Participate in activities that make you feel better, or that you used to enjoy before you began feeling depressed.
- Set realistic goals for yourself.
- Engage in mild exercise.
- Try to be with others and get support from them.
- Break up goals and tasks into smaller, more reachable ones.

Where Can I Find More Information about Depression?

National Institute of Mental Health Depression Fact Sheet: www.nimh .nih.gov/publicat/depression.cfm.

National Alliance on Mental Illness: www.nami.org.

National Center for Post-Traumatic Stress Disorder: www.ptsd.va.gov/.

*   *   *

SUICIDAL THOUGHTS AND SUICIDE

War experiences and war zone stress reactions, especially those caused by personal loss, can lead a depressed person to think about hurting or killing him- or herself. If you or someone you know is feeling this way, take it seriously, and get help. In the case of an emergency, call the National Suicide Prevention Lifeline at 800-273-TALK (8255) and press 1 for veterans.

Suicide Prevention

According to the DoD Suicide Prevention and Risk Reduction Committee's (SPARRC) Preventing Suicide Network, every year 30,000 Americans take their own lives. While the suicide rate for military members is substantially lower than for their civilian counterparts, it is still a significant cause of death for many of our military.

People commit suicide for reasons that are diverse and complex. Risk factors vary with age, gender, and race, and may occur in combination.

When records for over 100,000 veterans who served in Operations Enduring Freedom and Iraqi Freedom and sought treatment at a VA medical facility were reviewed, some similarities were discovered. The most common combination of diagnoses found was PTSD and depression.

These findings play into the known risk factors for suicide, including

- Stressful life events—when combined with depression or other risk factors. However, many people have stressful life events and are not at risk for suicide.
- A family history of mental disorder or substance abuse, especially if it includes violence—physical or sexual.
- A prior suicide attempt.
- A family history of suicide.
- Exposure to the suicidal behavior of others, such as family members, peers, or media figures.
- Depression, mental disorders, and substance abuse (more than 90 percent of the people who commit suicide have these risk factors).
- Having firearms in the home.
- Incarceration.

Most suicide attempts are not harmless bids for attention, but are expressions of extreme distress. A person who appears suicidal should not be left alone and needs immediate mental health treatment.

Most mental health problems were first identified during visits with primary care doctors, not with mental health professionals. Tell your doctor if you notice any of the following:

- Talking about wanting to hurt or kill yourself
- Trying to get pills, guns, or other things that you could use to harm yourself
- Talking or writing about death, dying, or suicide
- Hopelessness
- Rage, uncontrolled anger, seeking revenge
- Saying or feeling there's no reason for living
- Acting in a reckless or risky way
- Feeling trapped, like there's no way out

There are programs that can help you or your loved one get the help they need. Naturally, seek immediate medical attention (call 9-1-1) in the event of a suicide attempt.

MILITARY PROGRAMS

DoD Suicide Prevention and Risk Reduction Committee's (SPARRC) Preventing Suicide Network

The DoD SPARRC Preventing Suicide Network is a resource center aimed at providing authoritative and problem-specific information about suicide prevention. SPARRC aims to help military personnel, family, and friends who are concerned about someone who may be at risk for suicide so that they can locate tailored resources about suicide prevention. The program also educates the public, mental health clinicians, and other professionals about suicide prevention education and research, and it promotes active collaboration among professionals and consumers in all segments of suicide prevention treatment, policy, education, and research. The SPARRC website (see www.dcoe.health.mil) provides information on what to look for and what to do to help someone who you think may be dealing with thoughts of suicide. Up-to-date information is available so that you can become more educated about suicide and to see what researchers are currently doing. The site also provides service-specific resources that are listed below:

- Air Force—Air Force Suicide Prevention Program: afspp.afms.mil/.
- Army—U.S. Army Center for Health Promotion and Preventive Medicine, Suicide Prevention Program: chppm-www.apgea.army.mil/dhpw/Readi ness/suicide.aspx.
- Coast Guard—Coast Guard Suicide Prevention Program: www.uscg.mil/ worklife/suicide_prevention.asp.
- Marine Corps—Marine Corps Community Services Suicide Prevention Program: www.usmc-mccs.org/suicideprevent.
- Navy—Navy Suicide Prevention Program: www.npc.navy.mil/Command Support/SuicidePrevention.

GOVERNMENT SUICIDE PREVENTION PROGRAMS

National Suicide Prevention Lifeline

The National Suicide Prevention Lifeline is a national, 24-hour, toll-free suicide prevention service available to anyone in suicidal crisis who is seeking help. You can get help by dialing 800-273-TALK (8255), and then pressing 1 to be routed to the Veterans Hotline. This will then transfer you to the closest possible provider of mental health and suicide prevention services. To learn more about the Lifeline, local crisis centers, and other resources, go to www.suicidepreventionlifeline.org/Veterans/Default.aspx.

National Strategy for Suicide Prevention (NSSP)

The NSSP provides facts about suicide, recent publications, and resources designed to spread knowledge of the seriousness of suicides. A resource from their site can display state-specific suicide prevention programs. For more information, visit mentalhealth.samhsa.gov/suicideprevention.

National Institute of Mental Health (NIMH)

The Suicide Prevention section of the NIMH website contains information on statistics and prevention of suicide in the United States, resources that cover suicide and related mental illnesses, in addition to connections to ongoing clinical trials involved in suicide. To see this and more information, go to www.nimh.nih.gov/health/topics/suicide-prevention/index.shtml.

Centers for Disease Control and Prevention (CDC)

Suicide facts, risk factors, warning signs, and prevention strategies are described to provide you with a better understanding of how to recognize if you or someone you care for may be dealing with thoughts of suicide. To learn more, visit www.cdc.gov/ViolencePrevention/suicide/.

SUPPORT ORGANIZATIONS FOR THE PREVENTION OF SUICIDE

American Foundation for Suicide Prevention

The site offers assistance to people whose lives have been affected by suicide and offers support and opportunities to become involved in prevention. Learn more at www.afsp.org.

MedlinePlus

MedlinePlus provides information about warning signs and how to deal with them, as well as how to cope with suicide. Go to www.nlm.nih.gov/medlineplus/suicide.html.

National Association for People of Color Against Suicide (NOPCAS)

The NOPCAS website gives information on depression and other brain disorders, coping methods for survivors, and suicide prevention and intervention tips. Visit the website at www.nopcas.org/resources.

Depression Screening

The Live Your Life Well website from Mental Health America describes symptoms and treatments for depression and provides a free, confidential depression screening test. (Note: This screening test is not intended to provide a diagnosis for clinical depression, but may help identify any depressive symptoms and determine whether a further evaluation by a medical or mental health professional is necessary.) Check out the website at www.depression-screening.org.

Suicide Awareness Voices of Education (SAVE)

SAVE offers depression and suicide information, strategies for coping with loss, and resource links. Learn more at www.save.org.

Military Pathways

The Military Pathways program is designed for you to identify your own symptoms and access assistance for PTSD, depression, generalized anxiety disorder, alcohol use, and bipolar disorder before a problem becomes serious. Go to www.mentalhealthscreening.org/military/index.aspx for more information.

Centre for Suicide Prevention

This program of the Canadian Mental Health Association describes what to do if you or someone you care for is suicidal, provides resources for suicide prevention, and answers frequently asked questions about suicide. Visit the website at www.suicideinfo.ca/csp/go.aspx?tabid = 1.

Suicide Prevention Action Network (SPAN)

SPAN USA offers support to suicide survivors (those who have lost a loved one to suicide and those who have attempted suicide) and leverages to advance public policies that help prevent suicides. Check out the website at www.spanusa.org.

VIOLENCE AND ABUSE

Anger can sometimes turn into violence or physical abuse. It can also result in emotional and/or verbal abuse that can damage relationships. Abuse can take the form of threats, swearing, criticism, throwing things, conflict, pushing, grabbing, and hitting. If you were abused as a child, you are more at risk for abusing your partner or family members.

Here are a few warning signs that may lead to domestic violence:

- Controlling behaviors or jealousy
- Blaming others for problems or conflict
- Radical mood changes
- Verbal abuse such as humiliating, manipulating, confusing
- Self-destructive or overly risky actions; heated arguments

STRESS, TRAUMA, AND ALCOHOL AND DRUG ABUSE
A NATIONAL CENTER FOR PTSD FACT SHEET

Robyn D. Walser, Ph.D.

Drinking to Reduce Stress

Many military personnel experience stress related to their deployment, service, and return home. These quite natural stress reactions can range from mild to severe and may be either short-lived or persist for a very long time. One common approach to managing stress that seems a simple and easy solution is use of alcohol or drugs. Military personnel, like civilians, may use alcohol and drugs as a way to relax or reduce anxiety and other bad feelings. In some cases, alcohol and drugs are not only used to decrease stress but also to manage severe symptoms that can arise from a traumatic experience in the war zone. You might find yourself drinking or using drugs for a variety of reasons when under stress or after trauma, including to

- Help yourself sleep
- Decrease sadness
- Relax
- Help yourself be around others
- Decrease emotional pain
- Increase pleasurable experience
- "Drown" your worries
- Keep upsetting memories from coming to mind
- Escape present difficulties
- "Shake off" stress
- Calm anxiety

Becoming Dependent on Alcohol/Drugs

Initially, alcohol and drugs may seem to make things better. They may help you sleep, forget problems, or feel more relaxed. But any short-term benefit can turn sour fast. In the long run, using alcohol and drugs to cope with stress will cause a whole new set of very serious problems, as well as worsening the original problems that lead you to drink or use. Alcohol and drug abuse can cause problems with your family life, health, mental well-being, relationships, finances, employment, spirituality, and sense of self-worth.

Think about family impact as an example. It's difficult to create good relationships when you are regularly drunk or high. Being intoxicated decreases intimacy and creates an inability to communicate well. Family members can feel rejected by someone who is always under the influence. In addition, witnessing someone's behavior while under the influence can be distressing. Children may not understand the aggressive behavior, the shutting down, or the hiding out that can occur along with substance use. The fallout from an accident or an arrest can have a long-lasting impact on a family. Alcohol and drug problems are dangerous for loved ones, because they are often linked with family violence and driving while intoxicated.

When Is Use of Alcohol a Problem?

It is often hard to decide whether alcohol or drug use is becoming a problem. It can happen gradually, and sometimes it can be hard to notice by the person who is using. Here are things that people sometimes say to themselves to convince themselves that they do not have a problem. Do you recognize any?

- "I just drink beer (wine)."
- "I don't drink every day."
- "I don't use hard drugs."
- "I've never missed a day of work."
- "I'm not an alcoholic."
- "I don't need help, I can handle it."
- "I gave it up for three weeks last year—myself."

Alcohol or drug use can be considered a problem when it causes difficulties, even in minor ways. Here are some questions that you can ask yourself to see if you are developing a problem:

- Have friends or family members commented on how much or how often you drink?
- Have you have found yourself feeling guilty about your drinking or drug use?
- Have you found yourself drinking (using) more over time?
- Have you tried to cut down your alcohol (drug) use?
- Does your drinking (using drugs) ever affect your ability to fulfill personal obligations such as parenting or work?
- Do you drink (use) in situations that are physically dangerous such as driving or operating machinery while under the influence?
- Have you found that you need more alcohol (drug) to get the same effect?

If you find that you are answering yes to one or more of these questions, perhaps it is time to reevaluate your use, cut back, and seek help from friends, family, or a professional.

What to Do If Alcohol or Drugs Are Causing Problems

If you think that alcohol (drug) use has become (or is becoming) a problem for you, there are a number of things that you can do. First, recognize that you are not alone and that others are available to lend support. Second, find help. Getting help is the most useful tool in decreasing or stopping problem drinking or drug use, even if you have doubts about being able to quit or if you are feeling guilt about the problem. Call your health provider, contact a physician or therapist, call your local VA hospital, or contact your local Alcoholic's Anonymous for guidance in your recovery. These contacts can help you on the road to the life you want.

Listed below are some useful websites if you are looking for more information about alcohol and drug use or about how to get help.

Alcohol and Drug Abuse, Information and Resources: www.alcoholand drugabuse.com/.

National Institute on Alcohol Abuse and Alcoholism, Frequently Asked Questions: www.niaaa.nih.gov/FAQs/.

Substance Abuse Treatment Facility Locator: findtreatment.samhsa.gov/.

Alcoholics Anonymous: www.aa.org/.

*   *   *

SUBSTANCE ABUSE

It's common for troops to self-medicate. They drink or abuse drugs to numb out the difficult thoughts, feelings, and memories related to war zone experiences. While alcohol or drugs may seem to offer a quick solution, they actually lead to more problems. At the same time, a vast majority of people in our society drink. Sometimes it can be difficult to know if your drinking is actually a problem. Warning signs of an alcohol problem include

- Frequent excessive drinking
- Having thoughts that you should cut down
- Feeling guilty or bad about your drinking
- Others becoming annoyed with you or criticizing how much you drink
- Drinking in the morning to calm your nerves
- Problems with work, family, school, or other regular activities caused by drinking

SUBSTANCE ABUSE IN THE DEPLOYMENT ENVIRONMENT

R. Gregory Lande, DO FACN, Barbara A. Marin, Ph.D., and Josef I. Ruzek, Ph.D.

Comprehensive screening for substance abuse requires a three-part analysis. Health care providers should focus on behavior prior to deployment, during actual operations, and post deployment. Each situation deserves special, but brief and focused, screening.

For the vast majority of individuals the notice of impending deployment unleashes a myriad of cognitive and behavioral reactions. These reactions are generally mild and transient as the individuals' healthy coping mechanisms respond to the news. In a minority of cases the fear and uncertainty of the looming deployment precipitates a maladaptive response. Among this group, a fairly significant number will turn to substance abuse as a means of quelling the troubled pre-deployment emotions. In fact, current numbers estimate that roughly one-third of the American population meets criteria for problem drinking. Naturally, that figure would be higher among individuals manifesting varying degrees of behavioral difficulties.

A reasonable pre-deployment substance abuse screening strategy might begin with the general, but openly stated, recognition that a pending deployment normally elicits a wide range of emotions.

An innocuous screening interview might begin with a question such as,

"Individuals run the gamut from being excited to being petrified when notified of their deployment—what best characterizes your reaction?" Another question or two, based on the answer to the first question, could address the individual's coping style. For example, if an individual relates that the notice of deployment created a sense of anxiety and panic the health care provider might ask, "How are you handling your anxiety?" or "What makes you feel less stressed?" or "What plans are you making now that you have the notice of deployment?" Finally, a comment such as, "Some people find that drinking a bit more alcohol, smoking a few more cigarettes, or pouring some extra java helps relieve the stress—have you noticed this in yourself?" If this question prompts the individual to disclose tendencies in the direction of increased substance use, the heath care provider should then conduct a more formalized screen using the quantity-frequency questions followed, as appropriate, by the CAGE questions.

The quantity-frequency questions require three simple steps:

1. First ask, "On average, how many days a week do you drink alcohol?"
2. Then ask, "On a typical day when you drink, how many drinks do you have?"
3. Multiply the days of drinking a week times the number of drinks.

For example, an individual might report drinking a six-pack of beer Friday night and both weekend days. Using the above formula (3 days a week × 6 drinks per typical day) results in a score of 18. Any score exceeding 14 for men or 7 for women suggests an at-risk behavior. The next question in the quantity-frequency screen asks, "What is the maximum number of drinks you had on any given day since learning of your deployment?" A score exceeding 4 for men or 3 for women again suggests a potential problem with alcohol (Dawson, 2000).

Individuals identified by the quantity-frequency screen should next be asked the CAGE questions.

CAGE is an acronym for the following questions:
C—Have you ever felt that you should CUT down on your drinking?
A—Have people ANNOYED you by criticizing your drinking?
G—Have you ever felt bad or GUILTY about your drinking?

E—Have you ever had a drink first thing in the morning to steady your nerves or get rid of a hangover (i.e., as an EYE-OPENER)?

Individuals endorsing either three or four of the CAGE questions over the past year are most likely alcohol dependent. If the individual endorses one or two of the CAGE questions they may have current alcohol abuse. Combining the introductory screening comments with the quantity-frequency and CAGE questions can reliably predict 70–80 percent of individuals with alcohol abuse or dependence (Friedman et al., 2001).

The same screening tool can be adapted for illicit drug use. For example, the initial questions about the person's response to notification of deployment might uncover the use of marijuana. The health care provider can then ask quantity-frequency questions followed by the adapted CAGE.

Unfortunately, there are no predetermined cut-off scores for all the potential drugs of abuse, requiring the substitution of clinical judgment.

The screening tools described so far will help guide the care provider's thinking in determining the best intervention for the individual awaiting deployment. Persons with a CAGE score of 3 or 4 will require a more in-depth clinical evaluation focusing on alcohol- or drug-related disability. If further evaluation confirms the presence of alcohol or illicit drug dependence, the care provider should determine whether imminent deployment is in the best interest of the individual and the military mission. The care provider might recommend a diversion for treatment before deployment.

Individuals with a CAGE score of 1 or 2 will also require additional assessment. The focus here once again is on impairment but the range of possible interventions may not interfere with deployment. The care provider might determine for example that the spike in alcohol or drug consumption is temporary and will likely abate with a strong suggestion that abstinence or reduction is essential. Part of the decision making may center on the availability of alcohol or drugs in the theater of operations.

Typically forgotten in the abuse assessment are common legal products such a tobacco and caffeine. An increase in either prior to deployment may represent a soft warning signal that portends later problems. A substantial increase in the use of nicotine in the days leading up to deployment may be followed by a corresponding reduction once the individual arrives in the theater of operations. Many factors may promote the reduction, such as lack of availability or less free time, but the outcome will be the same. Nicotine withdrawal, most likely unrecognized, will produce irritability, dysphoria, and sleep disturbances.

Once the individual arrives in the theater of operations the stress of combat will be amplified by any preexisting, yet undetected, substance abuse problems. Two broad scenarios are possible. If the theater has easy access to drugs or alcohol then the pattern of abuse may continue or accelerate. If drug or alcohol acquisition is difficult, then the individual may experience symptoms of withdrawal. Clinicians in Iraq report that alcohol is easily accessible. Early on in the deployment, many were allowed to go to marketplaces in the cities where black market diazepam was cheap and readily available. Abuse of this drug decreased after trips to the marketplaces were discontinued for safety/security reasons.

The previously discussed substance abuse screening questions have just as much applicability in the combat zone as in the pre-deployment phase. The simplicity and accuracy of the screening questions are ideally suited to the triage environment of combat. Given the statistical frequency of substance abuse in the American population the care provider must strongly suspect any cognitive-behavioral symptoms arising in combat as the product of either ongoing use or withdrawal. Many of the signs and symptoms of alcohol withdrawal are easily misinterpreted. An individual presenting with autonomic hyperactivity, sleep difficulties, agitation, and anxiety may be suffering from withdrawal and not a combat-related acute stress disorder. Appropriate detection could prevent an unnecessary evacuation and lead instead to a brief in-theater detoxification.

Once again, care providers in the combat zone should screen for the common legal substances such as tobacco and caffeine. Prompt recognition of tobacco withdrawal symptoms could lead to a prescription for some form of nicotine replacement therapy. New products that help quit smoking such as bupropion and mecamylamine hold promise too. A subsequent period of observation may help distinguish the interaction between withdrawal effects and local stressors.

Any provider considering evacuating an individual from the theater of operations for a substance abuse disorder should carefully consider advising the individual about the likely treatment options and the impact on a military career. Hopefully, individuals evacuated from a combat zone for a substance abuse disorder will have been counseled regarding the value of treatment and the ultimate expectation that recovery will lead to future, productive military service, including possible redeployment to the combat zone. Care providers at the secondary or tertiary level facility can then assess the individual and recommend appropriate outpatient or inpatient treatment.

The clinician must consider the role of the military command regarding alcohol- and drug-related problems. A standing order prohibiting the use of any alcohol or illegal drugs exists in deployed environments. As a result, the military commander usually becomes involved when a soldier is identified in an alcohol- or drug-related incident. Commanders vary in their biases as how to handle these situations, but in general they try to balance their concerns for the individual soldier's medical/treatment needs with the need for unit discipline. Commanders often look for direction in balancing these legitimate concerns and usually appreciate input from mental health providers in making such decisions. At times, an inappropriately high level of tolerance of substance use or abuse occurs in some units. This may be more likely in National Guard or Reserve units. Some mental health clinicians in Iraq report that alcohol use in some units was prevalent to the degree that officers, noncommissioned officers (NCOs), and junior enlisted drink together. Though rare, such circumstances create significant challenges for proper unit functioning and for the effectiveness of mental health interventions.

Aside from screening for the common legal and illicit substances, the care provider in all phases of deployment should consider the role of herbal supplements, over-the-counter medications, and steroids. Another commonly neglected but easily screened issue involves the potential abuse of prescription medications.

Screening is also important in the post-deployment environment, where some individuals may resume previous problem drinking/drug use upon return to the United States or increase substance use as a means of coping with stress-related problems or attempting to manage traumatic stress reactions.

PTSD, depression, and alcohol and drug problems are often co-occurring in veterans. Both health and mental health providers should be alert to this and, as part of patient education, should inform returning veterans about safe drinking practices, discuss the relationship between traumatic stress reactions and substance abuse, and initiate preventive interventions to reduce drinking. Evidence suggests that substance abuse recovery is made more difficult by concurrent PTSD, and it is important to provide routine screening for PTSD in alcohol and drug treatment programs. When an individual is experiencing problems with both substance abuse and PTSD, it is important to address both disorders in an integrated fashion. Individuals should be helped to understand both problems and their relationship, and relapse prevention programming should address coping with traumatic stress symptoms without alcohol or drugs. Protocols for integrated treatment, such as the Seeking Safety trauma-relevant coping skills group intervention (Najavits, 2002), are now becoming available.

This brief clinical guide proposes a simple process, with proven accuracy, to screen individuals for substance abuse. This guide further suggests that care providers employ the screen in the three phases of pre-deployment, in the combat zone, and upon evacuation. The data gained at each juncture will help the clinician's decision-making process in clarifying the contribution of substance use to a muddled clinical picture, taking appropriate treatment steps, forestalling some unnecessary evacuations, and prompting the best match between the individual's needs and the military mission.

*   *   *

CASE STUDIES

The following case examples describe veterans who were treated at military and VA medical facilities. Information has been modified to protect patient identities.

Case 1

Specialist LR is a twenty-five-year-old single African American man who is an activated National Guardsman with four years of reserve service. He is a full-time college student and competitive athlete raised by a single mother in public housing. He has a history of minor assaults in school and his neighborhood and of exposure to street violence.

Initially trained in transportation, he was called to active duty and retrained as a military policeman to serve with his unit in Baghdad. He described enjoying the high intensity of his deployment and had become recognized by others as an informal leader because of his aggressiveness and self-confidence. He describes numerous exposures while performing convoy escort and security details. He reports coming under small arms fire on several occasions, witnessing dead and injured civilians and Iraqi soldiers and on occasion feeling powerless when forced to detour or take evasive action. He began to develop increasing mistrust of the operational environment, as the situation "on the street" seemed to deteriorate. He often felt that he and his fellow service personnel were placed in harm's way needlessly.

On a routine convoy mission, serving as driver for the lead HMMWV (Humvee), his vehicle was struck by an improvised explosive device (IED), showering him with shrapnel in his neck, arm, and leg. Another member of his vehicle was even more seriously injured. He described "kicking into autopilot," driving his vehicle to a safe location, and jumping out to do a battle damage assessment. He denied feeling much pain at that time. He was evacuated to the Combat Support Hospital (CSH) where he was treated and returned to duty (RTD) after several days despite requiring crutches and suffering chronic pain from retained shrapnel in his neck. He began to become angry at his command and doctors for keeping him in theater while he was unable to perform his duties effectively. He began to develop insomnia, hypervigilance, and a startle response. His initial dreams of the event became more intense and frequent and he suffered intrusive thoughts and flashbacks of the attack. He began to withdraw from his friends and suffered anhedonia, feeling detached from others, and he feared his future would be cut short. He was referred to a psychiatrist at the CSH who initiated supportive therapy and an SSRI.

After two months of unsuccessful rehabilitation for his battle injuries and worsening depressive and anxiety symptoms, he was evacuated to a stateside military medical center via a European medical center. He was screened for psychiatric symptoms and was referred for outpatient evaluation and management. He met DSM-IV criteria for acute PTSD and was offered medication management, supportive therapy, and group therapy, which he declined. He was treated with sertraline, trazodone, and clonazepam targeting his symptoms of insomnia, anxiety, and hyperarousal. Due to continued autonomic arousal, quetiapine was substituted for the trazodone and clonazepam for sleep and anxiety, and clonidine was started for autonomic symptoms. He responded favorably to this combination of medications. He avoided alcohol as he learned it would exacerbate symptoms. He was ambivalent about taking passes or convalescent leave to his home because of fears of being "different, irritated, or aggressive" around his family and girlfriend. After three months at the military medical center, he was sent to his demobilization site to await deactivation to his National Guard unit. He was referred to his local VA hospital to receive follow-up care.

Case 2

PV2 RJ is a twenty-six-year-old white female with less than twelve months of active duty service who was deployed to Iraq in September 2003. She reported excelling in high school but moved out of her house after becoming pregnant during her senior year. After graduating from high school on schedule, she worked at several jobs until she was able to become an x-ray assistant. She had been on her first duty assignment as an x-ray technician in Germany. As a single parent she attempted to make plans for her dependent five-year-old son. However, when notified of her impending deployment she needed to make hurried and unexpected care plans for her son.

Within a week of being deployed to Iraq the service member began experiencing depressed mood, decreased interest in activities, increased appetite, irritability, increased social isolation with passive suicidal ideations, and insomnia due to nightmares of the devil coming after her. She also began believing Saddam Hussein was the "Antichrist." In addition, she began experiencing command-directed auditory hallucination of the devil whispering to her that people in her unit were saying she was stupid and that she should make them shut up. At one time, the devil told her to throw things at them. Her guilt intensified as her wish to act on the voices increased. She also described seeing visual hallucinations of "monsters" that were making fun of her.

These symptoms intensified when she went from an in-processing point to her assignment in Iraq. They also worsened when she ruminated about the stresses of being in Iraq (bombs exploding, missing her son and family, disgust at other women who were seeking the attention of men). Of most concern, she was worried that she might not survive the deployment. When she was around people, she experienced palpitations, increased sweating, shaking, shortness of breath, abdominal cramping, and dizziness. In hopes of getting rid of her symptoms, especially the voices and monsters, she ingested Tylenol #3s she had obtained for a minor medical procedure. After confiding her symptoms to a military friend, RJ was referred for an evaluation and was evacuated out of Iraq to CONUS via Germany.

When she returned to CONUS, RJ also shared with the treatment team that in the week prior to deployment she believed she was drugged by a date and that he sexually assaulted her. RJ was hesitant to discuss the few memories she had of the incident, due to embarrassment. She denied any other previous traumatic events but she stated she distrusted men in general, as many men in her life had been unreliable or irresponsible. She admitted to occasional alcohol use but denied any drug use. Throughout the hospitalization, her greatest concern was being reunited with her son and leaving the military. She was treated with a combination of antidepressant and antipsychotic medications that resulted in improvement in her symptoms. Despite improvement, RJ underwent a Medical Evaluation Board for diagnoses of major depression with psychotic features and PTSD.

Case 3

SFC W is a forty-five-year-old divorced Operation Iraqi Freedom Reservist who was involved in a motor vehicle accident in Afghanistan in June 2003. SFC W suffered a lumbar burst fracture and had multiple surgical procedures with instrumentation and fusion at a European military medical center, which was complicated by a deep vein thrombosis.

SFC W was transferred through the aeromedical evacuation system to a stateside medical center where he was admitted as a non-battle injury for inpatient rehabilitation for spinal cord injury. SFC W's treatment plan consisted of a rehabilitation program involving physical and occupational therapy with goals of independent ambulation with an assistive device and to establish a bowel and bladder program. The Coumadin Clinic treated his deep vein thrombosis and he was evaluated by the Traumatic Brain Injury Program staff. Pain was controlled with MS Contin 15 mgm two times a day with oxycodone IR 5 mgm 1–2 tabs every 4–6 hours as needed for breakthrough pain and Ambien 10 mgm per day as needed for sleep problems. Other staff included in his care included nursing, social work, chaplain, Reserve Liason, and Medical Holding Company and Medical Board staff.

SFC W was followed by the Preventive Medicine Psychiatry Service (PMPS) in accordance with the service's Operation Iraqi Freedom Protocol. PMPS staff initially recommended beginning therapy with an SSRI such as sertraline at a starting dose of 25 mgm a day to address concerning symptoms, such as his increased startle response, emotional lability, and intrusive thoughts, which the staff thought could be prodromal for an acute stress disorder. PMPS staff also incorporated a combination of hypnotic and relaxation techniques to assist SFC W with sleep and pain-related problems. Staff recommended increasing sertraline to 50 mgm per day because he reported that he was continuing to be troubled by some memories of his accident.

Aside from the target symptoms that were addressed above, no other psychiatric issues were identified.

An initial Post-Deployment Health Assessment Tool (PDHAT) was completed during SFC W's hospital admission. He endorsed depressive symptoms at a level of 11 (a score of 10 or above indicates a potential concern) and endorsed symptoms consistent with PTSD (one intrusive symptom, two arousal symptoms, and three avoidance symptoms) at the level of a "little bit."

In June 2003, SFC W was transferred to the Spinal Cord Rehabilitation Program at a VA hospital. He was able to ambulate with the assistance of a walker; pain in his back and left leg was controlled with pain medicine, and his problems with a neurogenic bowel and bladder were well controlled with a daily bowel and bladder program. Additional traumatic brain testing and Coumadin regulation was requested.

Service personnel are contacted either telephonically or at the time of a follow-up visit to WRAMC and are assessed for PTSD, depression, alcohol usage, somatic complaints, days of poor physical and/or mental health and lost productivity, and satisfaction with health care.

SFC W could not be reached by phone until the six-month PDHAT follow-up. At that time he met criteria for major depression and had symptoms consistent with criteria for PTSD at the moderate level. He reported that he had lost twenty days of productivity due to physical and mental health problems. In addition, he reported problems with pain, sleep, sexual functioning, and the fact that he will never be the same again. He is able to ambulate with the assistance of a walker within his home and uses a wheelchair for outside excursions. He continues with a bowel program. His need to self-catheterize limits his visits outside the home. He is clinically followed at a local VA by psychiatry, neurology, spinal cord program, and physical therapy. He reported taking between twenty-five and thirty-five pills a day, including trazadone for sleep and sertraline 100 mgm po BID for treatment of depression and PTSD. He has accepted his functional limitations and is trying to adapt to the changes in his lifestyle. His support system is fairly good, he has a very supportive wife, his Reserve Unit is in contact with him, and he has attended social functions in recognition of returning Reservists. A request for case management services was submitted to the VA hospital to assist SFC W in understanding his medications, adapting to his functional limitations and understanding his long-term prognosis because of his spinal cord injury, and working through his PTSD symptoms to include trauma bereavement. Legal Assistance at WRAMC also assisted him with a claim for personal property lost as a result of his deployment to Iraq.

Prior to his deployment to Iraq, SFC W worked as a truck driver for a transportation company, a job that he will not be able to return to. His Medical Board is being processed, and he will then be eligible for both Army Medical Retirement and Veterans benefits.

Case 4

SGT P is a twenty-four-year-old married AD USA E5 who sustained penetrating wounds to his left arm, left ribs, and left leg in an improvised explosive device attack while in Iraq. Initially his wounds were treated in Kuwait, and he was MEDEVAC to a European military medical center where he underwent surgery to repair a fractured left ulna bone in summer 2003.

SGT P was air evacuated and admitted to the General Surgery Service at a stateside medical center. His recovery was uncomplicated and consisted of mostly rehabilitation and wound care.

He was initially followed by general surgery, vascular surgery, and orthopedics and was then discharged to Inpatient Physical Medicine and Rehabilitation (PMR) Service. While on the PMR Service, he progressed to ambulating hospital distances using a Lofstrand crutch and was moderately independent with activity of daily living. His pain was well controlled and he was discharged on Percocet 1–2 tabs every 4–6 hours, Motrin tabs 600 mgm 3x per day as needed, and Ambien 10 mgm every night for sleep.

SGT P was followed by the Preventive Medical Psychiatry Service in accordance with PMPS's Operation Iraqi Freedom Protocol. The PMPS staff initially met with him and offered support to set the milieu to establish a therapeutic alliance with him. His initial request was for assistance with contacting his command as he had not communicated with them since his injury and felt cut-off from his unit. During his first week in the hospital, Ambien 10 mgm po at bedtime was ordered to assist with sleep problems. He subsequently reported that Ambien was only minimally helping with his sleep problems and he was now experiencing nighttime "sweats." He denied experiencing any other arousal or intrusive symptoms and only endorsed limited avoidance of television news on OIF activities. PMPS staff discussed possible risks and benefits of starting propranol 20 mgm nightly to limit sympathetic discharge activity. SGT P agreed and was started on propranol 20 mgm at bedtime. Follow-up reports indicated that he was sleeping well and his autonomic hyperactivity had decreased. The use of pharmacotherapy interventions decreased his sleep disturbances and allowed him to be more open and responsive to psychotherapeutic interventions. PMPS staff also incorporated a combination of hypnotic and relaxation techniques to assist him with sleep and pain-related problems. Cognitive-behavioral therapy helped him understand how his traumatic experience may have altered his thoughts and interpretations of events and what effect the altered perceptions had on his emotions and behaviors. PMPS staff also assisted him in working through feelings of anger and reinforcing his coping strategies, identifying his strengths and assets.

The initial Post-Deployment Health Assessment Tool was completed during SGT P's inpatient admission, approximately sixteen days after his injury. At that time, he endorsed criteria for major depression and endorsed symptoms consistent with PTSD at the moderate level.

Two months after admission, SGT P was discharged from the hospital and placed on convalescent leave. He had follow-up appointments in the orthopedic and vascular clinics, physical therapy, and preventive medical psychiatry. He stayed at base hotel for the duration of his outpatient therapy.

PMPS staff followed SGT P on a regular basis during the course of the hospitalization and outpatient treatment, with visits ranging from one to three times per month. A combination of psychotherapy, hypnotherapy, and CBT interventions was provided. Ambien and propranol were not needed after the initial discharge medications were issued. He was able to regain control over the intrusive and arousal symptoms that he had been experiencing as a result of his deployment experience. Psychotherapeutic interventions assisted him in understanding the effect that his thoughts were having on his emotions and behavior and resulted in a substantial decrease in his endorsement of depressive symptoms (from 16 to 3 on the Pfizer, Prime MD Scale).

Service personnel are contacted either by telephone or in person at the time of follow-up and are assessed for PTSD, depression, alcohol usage, somatic complaints, days of poor physical and/or mental health, lost productivity, and satisfaction with health care. At the three-month PDHAT follow-up visit, SGT P endorsed a depressed mood but did not meet the full criteria for depression. He endorsed depressive symptoms at a level 12 (a score of 10 or above is of concern). PTSD symptoms were endorsed at a moderate level. Although, he reported nine days of poor mental and physical health during the previous month, he only reported two days of lost productivity due to poor mental or physical health. He reported excellent satisfaction with his health care. At the six-month PDHAT follow-up visit, he endorsed depressive symptoms at a level 3 and did not meet the criteria for depression. He endorsed mild intrusive symptoms but did not meet criteria for PTSD. SGT P has returned to a light duty status while he continues to recover from his injuries.

Health Care, Insurance, and Benefits

TRICARE PROGRAMS

TRICARE Prime is a managed-care option, similar to a civilian HMO (health maintenance organization). Prime is for active duty service members and available to other TRICARE beneficiaries. Active duty service members (ADSMs) are required to be enrolled in Prime; they must take action to enroll by filling out the appropriate enrollment form and submitting it to their regional contractor. There is no cost to the service member.

Other TRICARE beneficiaries may be eligible for Prime. Eligibility for any kind of TRICARE coverage is determined by the uniformed services. TRICARE manages the military health care program, but the services decide who is eligible to receive TRICARE coverage.

Prime enrollees receive most of their health care at a military treatment facility (MTF) and their care is coordinated by a primary care manager (PCM). Prime is not available everywhere.

Prime enrollees must follow some well-defined rules and procedures, such as seeking care, first, from the MTF. For specialty care, the Prime enrollee must receive a referral from his or her PCM and authorization from the regional contractor. Failure to do so could result in costly point of service (POS) option charges. Emergency care is not subject to POS charges.

TRICARE Prime Remote is the program for service members and their families who are on remote assignment, typically fifty miles from an MTF.

The TRICARE Overseas Program delivers the Prime benefit to ADSMs and their families in the three overseas areas: Europe, the Pacific, and Latin America/Canada. The TRICARE Global Remote program delivers the Prime benefit to ADSMs and families stationed in designated "remote" locations overseas.

TRICARE Standard is the basic TRICARE health care program, offering comprehensive health care coverage, for beneficiaries (not to include active duty members) not enrolled in TRICARE Prime. Standard does not require enrollment.

Standard is a fee-for-service plan that gives beneficiaries the option to see any TRICARE-certified/authorized provider (doctor, nurse-practitioner, lab, clinic, etc.). Standard offers the greatest flexibility in choosing a provider, but it will also involve greater out-of-pocket expenses for you, the patient. You also may be required to file your own claims.

Standard requires that you satisfy a yearly deductible before TRICARE cost sharing begins, and you will be required to pay copayments or cost shares for outpatient care, medications, and inpatient care.

TRICARE Extra can be used by any TRICARE-eligible beneficiary, who is not active duty, not otherwise enrolled in Prime, and not eligible for TRI-CARE for Life (TFL).

TRICARE Extra goes into effect whenever a Standard beneficiary chooses to make an appointment with a TRICARE network provider. Extra, like Standard, requires no enrollment and involves no enrollment fee.

TRICARE Extra is essentially an option for TRICARE Standard beneficiaries who want to save on out-of-pocket expenses by making an appointment with a TRICARE Prime network provider (doctor, nurse practitioner, lab, etc.). The appointment with the in-network provider will cost 5 percent less than it would with a doctor who is a TRICARE authorized or participating provider.

Also, the TRICARE Extra option-user can expect that the network provider will file all claims forms for him. The Standard beneficiary might have claims filed for him, but the non-network provider can decide to file on his behalf or not, on a case by case basis.

Under TRICARE Extra, because there is no enrollment, there is no Extra identification card. Your valid uniformed services ID card serves as proof of your eligibility to receive health care coverage from any TRICARE Prime provider.

TRICARE For Life (TFL) is a Medicare wraparound coverage available to Medicare-entitled uniformed service retirees, including retired guard members and reservists, Medicare-entitled family members and widows/widowers (dependent parents and parents-in-law are excluded), Medicare-entitled Congressional Medal of Honor recipients and their family members, and certain Medicare-entitled un-remarried former spouses.

To take advantage of TFL, you and your eligible family members' personal information and Medicare Part B status must be up to date in the Defense Enrollment Eligibility Reporting System (DEERS). You may update your information by phone (1-800-538-9552) or by visiting your nearest ID card issuing facility. Visit www.dmdc.osd.mil/rsl to locate the nearest ID card facility.

INSURANCE

Servicemembers' Group Life Insurance (SGLI)

SGLI is a program of low-cost group life insurance for servicemembers on active duty, ready reservists, members of the National Guard, members of the Commissioned Corps of the National Oceanic and Atmospheric Administration and the Public Health Service, cadets and midshipmen of the four service academies, and members of the Reserve Officer Training Corps.

SGLI coverage is available in $50,000 increments up to the maximum of $400,000. SGLI premiums are currently $.065 per $1,000 of insurance, regardless of the member's age. SGLI is highly recommended to be carried at all times, and recommended to be carried at maximum benefit during war time and/or during deployments.

Family Servicemembers' Group Life Insurance (FSGLI)

FSGLI is a program extended to the spouses and dependent children of members insured under the SGLI program. FSGLI provides up to a maximum of $100,000 of insurance coverage for spouses, not to exceed the amount of SGLI the insured member has in force, and $10,000 for dependent children. Spousal coverage is issued in increments of $10,000, at a monthly cost ranging from $.55 to $5.20 per increment.

Service members should contact their Personnel Support Center, Personnel Flight, Payroll, and/or Finance Office for SGLI and FSGLI premium payment information.

Traumatic Injury Protection under Servicemembers' Group Life Insurance (TSGLI)

Congress established the Servicemembers' Group Life Insurance Traumatic Injury Protection (TSGLI) program to offer emergency financial assistance to recovering service members who suffer severe traumatic injuries (on or off duty), or a qualifying loss as defined by regulation. TSGLI payments range from $25,000 to $100,000 in increments of $25,000. The Emergency Supplemental Appropriations Act for Defense, the Global War on Terror, and Tsunami Relief, 2005, signed by the president May 11, 2005, initiated the TSGLI program.

TSGLI provides financial assistance to recovering service members and their families through the period of recovery from a traumatic injury. This benefit is a tax-free, one-time, lump-sum payment per traumatic event and its purpose is not to serve as an ongoing income replacement. The amount the recovering service member receives varies depending on the injury.

TSGLI has been a rider to the Servicemembers' Group Life Insurance (SGLI) program since 2005. If you elect to receive SGLI, you automatically receive TSGLI coverage. An additional dollar to cover the costs of the program has been added to the monthly SGLI premium. A service member cannot decline TSGLI coverage as it is automatically included in the SGLI package.

TSGLI payments are designed to help traumatically injured service members and their families with financial burdens associated with recovering from a severe injury. TSGLI payments range from $25,000 to $100,000 based on the qualifying loss suffered. Every member who has SGLI also has TSGLI effective December 1, 2005. TSGLI coverage is automatic for those insured under basic SGLI and cannot be declined. The only way to decline TSGLI is to decline basic SGLI coverage. It is not recommended to decline basic SGLI coverage under any circumstances during a time of war.

The premium for TSGLI is a flat rate of $1 per month for most service members. Members who carry the maximum SGLI coverage of $400,000 will pay $29.00 per month for both SGLI and TSGLI.

To be eligible for payment of TSGLI, you must meet all of the following requirements:

- You must be insured by SGLI when you experience a traumatic event.
- You must incur a scheduled loss and that loss must be a direct result of a traumatic injury.
- You must have suffered the traumatic injury prior to midnight of the day that you separate from the uniformed services.

- You must suffer a scheduled loss within two years (730 days) of the traumatic injury.
- You must survive for a period of not less than seven full days from the date of the traumatic injury. (The seven-day period begins on the date and time of the traumatic injury, as measured by Zulu [Greenwich Meridian] time and ends 168 full hours later.)

To qualify for TSGLI, a recovering service member must be covered by one of the following groups:

- Members who incurred a qualifying traumatic injury between October 7, 2001, and November 30, 2005, while supporting OEF or OIF, or while deployed to a Combat Zone Tax Exclusion (CZTE) qualifying area
- Members who elected SGLI coverage and suffered a qualifying traumatic injury after December 1, 2005, regardless of their component (active, Reserve, or National Guard) or the location in which they incurred the traumatic injury

Qualifying traumatic injuries are those resulting from external force or violence or a condition that can be linked to a traumatic event. Such traumatic injuries must cause physical damage to the body. Qualifying injuries and payment amounts are listed in the TSGLI Schedule of Losses. You may view the complete schedule of losses at www.insurance.va.gov.

All qualifying losses that are a result of a traumatic injury must occur within 730 days of an identifiable traumatic event. There are certain circumstances under which a traumatic injury will not be covered by TSGLI. They include any injury

- Incurred prior to December 1, 2005, or between October 7, 2001, and November 30, 2005, but not in support of OEF/OIF or while under orders in a CZTE area
- Caused by a mental disorder or a mental or physical illness or disease (not including illness or disease caused by a wound infection, biological, chemical, or radiological weapon, or accidental ingestion of a contaminated substance)
- Incurred while attempting suicide, whether the service member was sane or insane

- Intentionally self-inflicted injury or any attempt to inflict such injury
- Incurred due to medical or surgical treatment of an illness whether the loss results directly or indirectly from that treatment
- Incurred while under the influence of an illegal or controlled substance unless administered or consumed on the advice of a doctor
- Incurred while committing or attempting to commit a felony

If you feel that you qualify for TSGLI, you can obtain a TSGLI claim form by visiting www.insurance.va.gov/sglisite/TSGLI/TSGLI.htm or contacting the TSGLI point of contact for your service on the following list:

TSGLI Army
800-237-1336, press option 2 for TSGLI, or TSGLI@conus.army.mil
www.hrc.army.mil/site/crsc/tsgli/index.html

Army National Guard
703-607-5851, or raymond.holdeman@ng.army.mil
www.hrc.army.mil/site/crsc/tsgli/index.html

TSGLI Navy
800-368-3202, or MILL_TSGLI@navy.mil
www.npc.navy.mil/CommandSupport/CasualtyAssistance/TSGLI/

TSGLI Marine Corps
877-216-0825 or 703-432-9277, or t-sgli@usmc.mil
www.manpower.usmc.mil/portal/page?_pageid = 278,3206641&
   _dad;cqportal&_schema = PORTAL

TSGLI Air Force
210-565-3505, or afpc.casualty@randolph.af.mil
Air Reserves
800-525-0102 ext 227
Air National Guard
703-607-1239

TSGLI Coast Guard
202-475-5391, or terrence.w.walsh@uscg.mil

Exceptional Family Member Program (EFMP)

The EFMP is a mandatory enrollment program, based on carefully defined rules. EFMP works with other military and civilian agencies to provide comprehensive and coordinated medical, educational, housing, community support, and personnel services to families with special needs. EFMP enrollment works to ensure that needed services are available at the receiving command before the assignment is made.

An Exceptional Family Member is a dependent, regardless of age, who requires medical services for a chronic condition, receives ongoing services from a specialist, has behavioral health concerns/social problems/psychological needs, receives education services provided on an individual education program (IEP), or a family member receiving services provided on an individual family services plan (IFSP). The military member is responsible for contacting the EFMP service office on base and enrolling family members who meet the above description, and for maintaining any and all updates to the EFMP paperwork. The EFMP program also has a coordinator who may be knowledgeable about local, military, or related community services that may benefit the EFMP family member(s).

VA HEALTH CARE BENEFITS

Basic Eligibility

If you served in the active military, naval, or air service and are separated under any condition other than dishonorable, you may qualify for VA health care benefits. If you are a member of the Reserves or National Guard who was called to active duty (other than for training only) by a federal order and completed the full period for which you were called or ordered to active duty, you may be eligible for VA health care as well.

Minimum Duty Requirements

If you enlisted after September 7, 1980, or entered active duty after October 16, 1981, you must have served twenty-four continuous months or the full period for which you were called to active duty in order to be eligible. This minimum duty requirement may not apply to you if you were discharged for a disability incurred or aggravated in the line of duty.

Enrollment (VA Form 10-10 EZ)

To apply for VA health care, you must complete VA Form 10-10 EZ, Application for Health Benefits, which may be obtained from any VA health care facility or regional benefits office, online at https://www.1010ez.med.va .gov/sec/vha/1010ez/ or by calling 877-222-VETS (8387). Many military treatment facilities have VA representatives on staff who can also help you with this request.

If you fall into one of the following categories, you are not required to enroll using VA Form 10-10 EZ to receive care from VA, but VA suggests that you still do enroll because it allows their staff to better plan health resources for all veterans if they can identify how many people are eligible for care. The categories are

- Veterans with a service-connected disability of 50 percent or more
- Veterans seeking care for a disability the military determined was incurred or aggravated in the line of duty, but which VA has not yet rated, within twelve months of discharge
- Veterans seeking care for a service-connected disability only
- Veterans seeking registry examinations (Ionizing Radiation, Agent Orange, Gulf War/Operation Iraqi Freedom and Depleted Uranium)

Service Disabled Veterans

If you are 50 percent or more disabled from service-connected conditions, unemployable due to service-connected conditions, or receiving care for a service-connected disability, you will receive priority in scheduling of hospital or outpatient medical appointments.

Combat Veterans

If you were discharged from active duty on or after January 28, 2003, you are eligible for enhanced enrollment placement for five years after the date you leave service. If you served in combat after November 11, 1998, were discharged from active duty before January 28, 2003, and apply for enrollment on or after January 28, 2008, you are eligible for this enhanced enrollment benefit through January 27, 2011. You may also be eligible for enhanced enrollment if you were an activated Reservist or member of the National Guard who served on active duty in a theater of combat operations after November 11, 1998, and left service under any conditions other than dishonorable. If you enroll with VA under this "Combat Veteran" authority, you keep your enrollment eligibility even after their five-year post-discharge period ends. At the end of the post-discharge period, VA will reassess your information (including all applicable eligibility factors) and make a new enrollment decision.

BEHAVIORAL HEALTH CARE SERVICES

Some people experience effects from the stress of combat that don't go away without help, or may even get worse over time. You may suffer nightmares, flashbacks, difficulty sleeping, and feeling emotionally numb. These symptoms can significantly impair your daily life. You may also feel depressed, begin to abuse alcohol or drugs, have problems with memory and understanding, and have difficulty dealing with social or family situations.

Mental and behavioral health care is also a TRICARE benefit. TRICARE will cover care that is medically or psychologically necessary in both outpatient and inpatient settings. Your first eight behavioral health outpatient visits per fiscal year do not require prior authorization from TRICARE.

8

Families

FAMILY INVOLVEMENT IN CARE

The primary source of support for the returning soldier is likely to be his or her family. We know from veterans of the Vietnam War that there can be a risk of disengagement from family at the time of return from a war zone. We also know that emerging problems with ASD and PTSD can wreak havoc with the competency and comfort the returning soldier experiences as a partner and parent. While the returning soldier clearly needs the clinician's attention and concern, that help can be extended to include his or her family as well. Support for the veteran and family can increase the potential for the veteran's smooth immediate or eventual reintegration back into family life and reduce the likelihood of future more damaging problems.

Outpatient Treatment

If the veteran is living at home, the clinician can meet with the family and assess with them their strengths and challenges and identify any potential risks. Family and clinician can work together to identify goals and develop a treatment plan to support the family's reorganization and return to stability in coordination with the veteran's work on his or her own personal treatment goals.

If one or both partners are identifying high tension or levels of disagreement, or the clinician is observing that their goals are markedly incompatible, then issues related to safety need to be assessed and plans might need to be made that support safety for all family members. Couples who have experienced domestic violence and/or infidelity are at particularly high risk and in need of more immediate support. When couples can be offered a safe forum for discussing, negotiating, and possibly resolving conflicts, that kind of clinical support can potentially help to reduce the intensity of the feelings that can become dangerous for a family. Even support for issues to be addressed by separating couples can be critically valuable, especially if children are involved and the parents anticipate future coparenting.

Residential Rehabilitation Treatment

Inpatient hospitalization could lengthen the time returning personnel are away from their families, or it could be an additional absence from the family for the veteran who has recently returned home. It is important to the ongoing support of the reuniting family that clinicians remain aware that their patient is a partner and/or parent. Family therapy sessions, in person or by phone if geographical distance is too great, can offer the family a forum for working toward meeting their goals. The potential for involving the patient's family in treatment will depend on their geographic proximity to the treatment facility. Distance can be a barrier, but the family can still be engaged through conference phone calls, or visits as can be arranged.

FOR THE FAMILY

TBI of any severity can disrupt families, in no small part because of family members' changing roles in response to the patient's difficulties, even if these problems ultimately improve. Immediate family involvement and education about the course of illness is crucial, and ongoing attention should be paid to family needs as time passes. Supporting families can improve outcomes by ensuring that the patient's recovery is not hampered by a deteriorating family situation. Many providers will not have the time or expertise to include families in all phases of treatment; again, clinicians should not hesitate to seek out expertise and support groups early in the course of illness.

WAR-ZONE-RELATED STRESS REACTIONS: WHAT FAMILIES NEED TO KNOW A NATIONAL CENTER FOR PTSD FACT SHEET

Julia M. Whealin, Ph.D.

Military personnel in war zones frequently have serious reactions to their traumatic war experiences. Sometimes the reactions continue after they return home. Ongoing reactions to war zone fear, horror, or helplessness connected with post-traumatic stress can include:

- Nightmares or difficulty sleeping
- Unwanted distressing memories or thoughts
- Anxiety and panic
- Irritability and anger
- Emotional numbing or loss of interest in activities or people
- Problem alcohol or drug use to cope with stress reactions

How Traumatic Stress Reactions Can Affect Families

Stress reactions in a returning war veteran may interfere with the ability to trust and be emotionally close to others. As a result, families may feel emotionally cut off from the service member. The veteran may feel irritable and have difficulty with communication, making him or her hard to get along with. He or she may experience a loss of interest in family social activities. The veteran may lose interest in sex and feel distant from his or her spouse. Traumatized war veterans often feel that something terrible may happen "out of the blue" and can become preoccupied with trying to keep themselves and family members safe.

Just as war veterans are often afraid to address what happened to them, family members also may avoid talking about the trauma or related problems. They may avoid talking because they want to spare the veteran further pain, or because they are afraid of his or her reaction. Family members may feel hurt, alienated, or discouraged because the veteran has not overcome the effects of the trauma and may become angry or feel distant from the veteran.

The Important Role of Families in Recovery

The primary source of support for the returning soldier is likely to be his or her family. Families can help the veteran avoid withdrawal from others. Families can provide companionship and a sense of belonging, which can help counter feelings of separateness and difference from other people. They can provide practical and emotional support for coping with life stressors.

If the veteran agrees, it is important for family members to participate in treatment. It is also important to talk about how the post-trauma stress is affecting the family and what the family can do about it. Adult family members should also let their loved ones know that they are willing to listen if the service member would like to talk about war experiences. Family members should talk with treatment providers about how they can help in the recovery effort.

Self-Care Suggestions for Families

- Become educated about PTSD.
- Take time to listen to all family members and show them that you care.
- Spend time with other people. Coping is easier with support from caring others, including extended family, friends, church, or other community groups.
- Join or develop a support group.
- Take care of yourself. Family members frequently devote themselves totally to those they care for, and in the process, neglect their own needs. Watch your diet, exercise, and get plenty of rest. Take time to do things that feel good to you.
- Try to maintain family routines, such as dinner together, church, or sports outings.

*   *   *

HOMECOMING AFTER DEPLOYMENT: DEALING WITH CHANGES AND EXPECTATIONS
A NATIONAL CENTER FOR PTSD FACT SHEET

Ilona Pivar, Ph.D.

With deployment comes change. Knowing what to expect and how to deal with changes can make homecoming more enjoyable and less stressful. Below are some hints you might find helpful.

Expectations for Service Personnel

- You may miss the excitement of the deployment for a while.
- Some things may have changed while you were gone.
- Face-to-face communication may be hard at first.
- Sexual closeness may also be awkward at first.
- Children have grown and may be different in many ways.
- Roles may have changed to manage basic household chores.
- Spouses may have become more independent and learned new coping skills.
- Spouses may have new friends and support systems.
- You may have changed in your outlook and priorities in life.
- You may want to talk about what you saw and did. Others may seem not to want to listen. Or you may not want to talk about it when others keep asking.

Expectations for Spouses

Your partner

- May have changed.
- May be used to the open spaces of the field, may feel closed in.
- May be overwhelmed by noise and confusion of home life.
- May be on a different schedule of sleeping and eating (jet lag).
- May wonder if he or she still fits into the family.
- May want to take back all the responsibilities he or she had before deployment.
- May feel hurt when young children are slow to hug them.

What Children May Feel

- Babies less than one year old may not know you and may cry when held.
- Toddlers (1–3 years) may hide from you and be slow to come to you.
- Preschoolers (3–5 years) may feel guilty over the separation and be scared.
- School age (6–12 years) may want a lot of your time and attention.
- Teenagers (13–18 years) may be moody and may appear not to care.
- Any age may feel guilty about not living up to your standards.
- Some may fear your return ("Wait until mommy/daddy gets home!").
- Some may feel torn by loyalties to the spouse who remained.

*   *   *

**HOMECOMING AFTER DEPLOYMENT: TIPS FOR REUNION
A NATIONAL CENTER FOR PTSD FACT SHEET**

Pamela J. Swales, Ph.D.

Reunion is part of the deployment cycle and is filled with joy and stress. The following tips can help you have the best possible reunion.

Tips for Service Personnel

- Support good things your family has done.
- Take time to talk with your spouse and children.
- Make individual time for each child and your spouse.
- Go slowly when reestablishing your place in the family.
- Be prepared to make some adjustments.
- Romantic conversation can lead to more enjoyable sex.
- Make your savings last longer.

- Take time to listen and to talk with loved ones.
- Go easy on partying.

Tips for Spouses for Reunion
- Avoid scheduling too many things.
- Go slowly in making adjustments.
- You and your soldier may need time for yourself.
- Remind soldier he or she is still needed in the family.
- Discuss splitting up family chores.
- Stick to your budget until you've had time to talk it through.
- Along with time for the family, make individual time to talk.
- Be patient with yourself and your partner.

Tips for Reunion with Children
- Go slowly. Adapt to the rules and routines already in place.
- Let the child set the pace for getting to know you again.
- Learn from how your spouse managed the children.
- Be available to your child, both with time and with your emotions.
- Delay making changes in rules and routines for a few weeks.
- Expect that the family will not be the same as before you left; everyone has changed.
- Focus on successes with your children; limit your criticisms.
- Encourage children to tell you about what happened during the separation.
- Make individual time for each child and your spouse.

*   *   *

CAREGIVER SUPPORT
Your military spouse, son, or daughter may have an injury or illness, and, as a result, may require a considerable amount of care once released from the hospital. Many family members of recovering service members have found themselves in this role. Sometimes this role is temporary while the service member recovers. Other times, as is sometimes the case with traumatic brain injuries, you may be in the role of caregiver for a much longer time.

As a new caregiver, you may be concerned about your abilities to handle the task, wondering if you can cope with the change in your role, fearful of what is ahead, and you may be mourning the loss of the way things were before the injury or illness. You may feel overwhelmed and not know where to turn for help.

There are a variety of resources that can help you. You are not alone. As a caregiver, you may be relied upon to help your loved one with a broad range of activities, including cooking, eating, bathing, and dressing. You may need to take care of paying his or her bills and making medical decisions. A variety of services are available to help you assist a disabled service member or veteran.

Assessing Your Needs

In order to know what assistance you need, you may find it helpful to ask yourself the following questions:

- What type of help does my husband/wife/son/daughter need in order to live as independently as possible? (Consider the following options: companionship, housekeeping, grocery shopping, and transportation to the military treatment facility.)
- When do you need help?
- What help can be provided?
- How much money is available to pay for outside resources? Do you have additional insurance to help offset the cost of these services?
- Are any friends or family willing to pitch in? What help have they offered?

Caregiving Can Take a Toll on You

Research suggests that the physical and emotional demands on caregivers put them at greater risk for health problems:

- Caregivers are more at risk for infectious diseases, such as colds and flu, and chronic diseases, such as heart problems, diabetes, and cancer.
- Depression is twice as common among caregivers compared to noncaregivers.

Caregivers and Depression

If you find yourself feeling sad, alone, overwhelmed, or angry, you may be experiencing depression. It's not unusual for caregivers to experience mild to more severe depression.

While the caregivers do everything they can to give the best possible care to their injured loved one, they often place their own physical and emotional needs second, third—even last. After a while, this can cause anger, sadness, isolation, and exhaustion. Once these feeling are identified, guilt often results. Thoughts like, "How can I blame him? It's not his fault that he was injured," or "She's my 'baby' and needs me. How can I put my needs ahead of hers?" can cause monumental guilt, driving you to work through the negative feelings and, once again, put your needs after the injured person's needs.

Everyone has negative feelings, but if they don't go away, or if they leave you drained of energy and you find yourself angry at your loved one, or crying all the time, they may be signs that you are depressed. Ignoring the feelings will not make them go away.

Symptoms of Depression

The symptoms of depression are different for everyone and only a mental health care professional is qualified to tell you if you are clinically depressed. There are symptoms that may indicate depression. Some are listed below:

- Difficulty staying focused
- Significant weight loss or gain from a change in eating habits
- Sleeping much more or having difficulty sleeping
- Constant fatigue
- Lack of interest in the activities and people you once enjoyed
- Feelings of hopelessness
- Thoughts of hurting yourself
- Thoughts of killing yourself
- Constant disorders (headache, stomach ache, etc.) that do not respond to treatment

It's essential to get help for your depression. Without assistance, your quality of life will continue to decline.

How You Can Combat Depression

First, you should consult with a trained health or mental health professional. If you think that you are depressed, a good place to get help is to start with your family doctor. If you feel uncomfortable saying that you think you are depressed, tell your health professional that you "feel blue" or "feel down." They will know what to ask. Be prepared to answer questions like

- Why do you think you feel this way?
- When did the symptoms start?
- How long have you felt this way?
- How often do you use alcohol or drugs to feel better?
- Do you have family members who suffer from depression?
- Do you have a friend or someone with whom you can confide?

Besides the health professional's treatment, there are ways you can help yourself. In no way are these suggestions meant to be replacements for professional care. But taking care of yourself in the following ways may help ease some of your depression.

- Set realistic goals. Examples might include going to bed thirty minutes earlier; loading the dishwasher in the morning; making a simple, quick dinner rather than a more elaborate meal.
- Try to be with other people—confide in a friend.
- Do something enjoyable—work in thirty minutes of exercise, go to a movie, meet a friend for coffee.
- Break larger tasks into smaller ones and accomplish what you can.
- Try to think positive thoughts.
- Let your friends and family help you.
- Eat balanced meals.

Help is always as close as your friends, family, and the network of those in a similar situation. Remember, there are others who are in a similar situation as you. Reach out to them through support groups, in person, or online. You may find that sharing experiences will help you in a number of ways.

COMMUNITY CARE OPTIONS

Community care programs and services, along with eligibility requirements, vary in different states, counties, and communities. Many of these agencies and organizations are located on the National Resource Directory website. Informal support offered by friends, family, religious communities, local organizations, neighbors, and others can share the responsibilities of care giving, including household chores, provide emotional support for you and your loved one, and help the recovering service member maintain a healthy level of social and recreational activity.

In this case, making a list of your helpers and their phone numbers will be an invaluable source of support for routine help or in times of emergency.

Information and referral helps you by identifying your local resources. See the resources in chapter 11 for organizations that provide information and referral as part of their services.

FOR THE WARRIOR: BACK HOME WITH FAMILY

Common Experiences and Expectations You May Face

There is usually a "honeymoon" phase shortly after demobilization, but honeymoons come to an end. You and members of your family have had unique experiences and have changed. You'll need to get to know each other again and appreciate what each other went through. Very likely, you'll need to renegotiate some of your roles. You will need time to rebuild intimacy and learn how to rely on one another again for support.

In addition, your interests may have changed. You may need to reexamine future plans, dreams, and expectations. You and your family will also need to reexamine common goals.

When you return to life at home, you may

- Feel pressured by requests for time and attention from family, friends, and others
- Be expected to perform home, work, and school responsibilities, or care for children before you are ready
- Find that your parents are trying to be too involved or treat you like a child again
- Face different relationships with children who now have new needs and behaviors
- Be confronted by the needs of partners who have had their own problems

Financial Concerns

You may have financial issues to handle when you return home.

- Be careful not to spend impulsively.
- Seek assistance if making ends meet is hard due to changes in income.

Work Challenges

Readjusting to work can take time.

- You may feel bored, or that you find no meaning in your former work.
- You may have trouble finding a job.

If You Have Children

Children react differently to deployment depending on their age. They can cry, act out, be clingy, withdraw, or rebel. To help, you can

- Provide extra attention, care, and physical closeness.
- Understand that they may be angry and perhaps rightly so.
- Discuss things. Let kids know they can talk about how they feel. Accept how they feel and don't tell them they should not feel that way.
- Tell kids their feelings are normal. Be prepared to tell them many times.
- Maintain routines and plan for upcoming events.

Common Reactions You May Have That Will Affect
Family-and-Friend Relationships

At first, many service members feel disconnected or detached from their partner and/or family. You may be unable to tell your family about what happened. You may not want to scare them by speaking about the war. Or maybe you think that no one will understand. You also may find it's hard to express positive feelings. This can make loved ones feel like they did something wrong or are not wanted anymore. Sexual closeness may also be awkward for a while. Remember, it takes time to feel close again.

When reunited with family, you may also feel

- Mistrusting: During your deployment you trusted only those closest to you, in your unit. It can be difficult to begin to confide in your family and friends again.
- Overcontrolling or overprotective: You might find that you're constantly telling the kids "Don't do that!" or "Be careful, it's not safe!" Rigid discipline may be necessary during wartime, but families need to discuss rules and share in decisions.

- Short tempered: More conflicts with others may be due to poor communication and/or unreasonable expectations.

BATTLEMIND

In the past few years, the military has made a greater effort to prepare troops for reentry to civilian life. The Army has designed a post-deployment training experience called BATTLEMIND. The program helps service members understand how a wartime mind-set is useful at war but not at home.

Each letter in BATTLEMIND stands for a mind-set. For example:

The "B" stands for Buddies versus withdrawal. When deployed, buddies are the only ones you talk with, but at home this can lead you to withdraw from family and friends. Take time to reconnect.

The final "D" stands for Discipline, which is essential in the military but problematic if applied too strictly with family. Your thirteen-year-old daughter might not obey orders in the same way you are used to!

Each branch of the military has its own version of the BATTLEMIND approach. For more information, visit www.battlemind.army.mil.

Traumatic war experiences often cause many of the following kinds of (often temporary) reactions.

Unwanted Remembering or Reexperiencing

Almost all veterans experience difficulty controlling distressing memories of war. Although these memories are upsetting, on the positive side, the memories provide an opportunity for the person to make sense of what happened and gain mastery over the event. The experience of these memories can include

- Unwanted distressing memories as images or other thoughts
- Feeling like it is happening again (flashbacks)

- Dreams and nightmares
- Distress and physical reactions (e.g., heart pounding, shaking) when reminded of the trauma

Physical Activation or Arousal

The body's fight or flight reaction to a life-threatening situation continues long after the event is over. It is upsetting to feel like your body is overreacting or out of control. However, on the positive side, these fight-or-flight reactions help prepare a person in a dangerous situation for quick response and emergency action. Signs of continuing physical activation, common following participation in war, can include

- Difficulty falling or staying asleep
- Irritability, anger, and rage
- Difficulty concentrating
- Being constantly on the lookout for danger (hypervigilance)
- Being startled easily, for example, when hearing a loud noise (exaggerated startle response)
- Anxiety and panic

Shutting Down: Emotional Numbing

When overwhelmed by strong emotions, the body and mind sometimes react by shutting down and becoming numb. As a result, veterans may have difficulty experiencing loving feelings or feeling some emotions, especially when upset by traumatic memories. Like many of the other reactions to trauma, this emotional numbing reaction is not something the veteran is doing on purpose.

Active Avoidance of Trauma-Related Thoughts and Feelings

Painful memories and physical sensations of fear can be frightening, so it is only natural to try to find ways to prevent them from happening. One way that most veterans do this is by avoiding anything—people, places, conversations, thoughts, emotions and feelings, physical sensations—that might act as a reminder of the trauma. This can be very helpful if it is used once in a while (e.g., avoiding upsetting news or television programs). But when avoidance is used too much, it can have two big negative effects.

First, it can reduce veterans' abilities to live their lives and enjoy themselves, because they can become isolated and limited in where they go and what they do. Second, avoiding thoughts and emotions connected with the trauma may reduce veterans' abilities to recover from it. It is through thinking about what happened, and particularly through talking about it with trusted others, that survivors may best deal with what has happened. By constantly avoiding thoughts, feelings, and discussions about the trauma, this potentially helpful process can be short-circuited.

Depression

Most persons who have been traumatized experience depression. Feelings of depression then lead a person to think very negatively and feel hopeless. There is a sense of having lost things: one's previous self (I'm not the same person I was), a sense of optimism and hope, self-esteem, and self-confidence. With time, and sometimes with the help of counseling, the trauma survivor can regain self-esteem, self-confidence, and hope. It is important to let others know about feelings of depression and, of course, about any suicidal thoughts and feelings, which are sometimes a part of feeling depressed.

Self-blame, Guilt, and Shame

Many veterans, in trying to make sense of their traumatic war experiences, blame themselves or feel guilty in some way. They may feel bad about something(s) they did or didn't do in the war zone. Feelings of guilt or self-blame cause much distress and can prevent a person from reaching out for help. Therefore, even though it is hard, it is very important to talk about guilt feelings with a counselor or doctor.

Interpersonal Problems

Not surprisingly, the many changes noted above can affect relationships with other people. Trauma may cause difficulties between a veteran and his or her partner, family, friends, or coworkers. Particularly in close relationships, the emotional numbing and feeling of disconnection that are common after traumatic events may create distress and drive a wedge between the survivor and his or her family or close friends. The survivor's avoidance of different kinds of social activities may frustrate family members. Sometimes this avoidance results in social isolation that hurts relationships.

Others may respond in ways that worsen the problem rather than help recovery. They may have difficulty understanding, become angry with the veteran, communicate poorly, and fail to provide support. Partners and families need to participate in treatment; by learning more about traumatic stress, they can often become more understanding of the veteran and feel more able to help. Some kinds of traumatic experiences (e.g., sexual assault) can make it hard to trust other people.

These problems in relationships are upsetting. Just as the veteran needs to learn about trauma and its effects, people who are important to him or her also need to learn more. As the survivor becomes more aware of trauma reactions and how to cope with them, he or she will be able to reduce the harm they cause to relationships.

Physical Symptoms and Health Problems

Because many traumas result in physical injury, pain is often part of the experience of survivors. This physical pain often causes emotional distress, because in addition to causing pain and discomfort, the injury also reminds them of their trauma. Because traumas stress the body, they can sometimes affect physical health, and survivors may experience stress-related physical symptoms such as headaches, nausea or other stomach problems, and skin problems. The veteran with PTSD will need to care for his or her health, seek medical care when appropriate, and inform the doctor or nurse about his or her traumas, in order to limit the effects of the trauma.

Aggressive driving is also extremely common among service members returning from conflicts in the Middle East. Although you want to drive when you get back, you need to use extra caution. This is particularly true if you're feeling edgy or upset.

HEALTHY COPING FOR COMMON REACTIONS TO TRAUMA

With homecoming, you may need to relearn how to feel safe, comfortable, and trusting with your family. You must get to know one another again. Good communication with your partner, children, parents, siblings, friends, coworkers, and others is the key. Give each other the chance to understand what you have been through. When talking as a family, be careful to listen to one another. Families work best when there is respect for one another and a willingness to be open and consider alternatives.

Tips for Feeling Better

It's fine for you to spend some time alone. But if you spend too much time alone or avoid social gatherings, you will be isolated from family and friends. You need the support of these people for a healthy adjustment. You can help yourself to feel better by

- Getting back to regular patterns of sleep and exercise
- Pursuing hobbies and creative activities
- Planning sufficient R&R and intimate time
- Trying relaxation techniques (meditation, breathing exercises) to reduce stress
- Learning problems to watch out for and how to cope with them
- Striking a balance between staying connected with former war buddies and spending individual time with your partner, kids, other family members, and friends
- Communicating more than the "need-to-know" bare facts
- Talking about your war zone experiences at a time and pace that feels right to you
- Not drinking to excess, or when you're feeling depressed, or to avoid disturbing memories. Drink responsibly, or don't drink
- Creating realistic workloads for home, school, and work

Steps to Assuming Normal Routines

Soon after your return, plan to have an open and honest discussion with your family about responsibilities. You all need to decide how they should be split up now that you're home. It's usually best to take on a few tasks at first and then more as you grow accustomed to being home. Be willing to compromise so that both you and your family members feel that needs are understood and respected.

Try to reestablish a normal sleep routine as quickly as possible. Go to bed and get up at the same time every day. Do not drink to help yourself sleep. You might try learning some relaxation techniques, such as deep breathing, yoga, or meditation.

Steps to Controlling Anger

Recognize and try to control your angry feelings. Returning service members don't always realize how angry they are. In fact, you may only recognize your emotion when someone close to you points it out. You can help control your anger by

- Counting to ten or twenty before reacting
- Figuring out the cues or situations that trigger your anger so you can be better prepared
- Learning relaxation techniques (breathing, yoga, meditation)
- Learning ways to deal with irritation and frustration and how not to be provoked into aggressive behavior
- Walking away
- Thinking about the ultimate consequences of your responses
- Writing things down
- Learn tips to controlling anger

Important Points to Remember

- Readjusting to civilian life takes time—don't worry that you're experiencing some challenges. Find solutions to these problems. Don't avoid.
- Take your time adding responsibilities and activities back into your life.
- Reconnect with your social supports. This may be the last thing you feel like doing, but do it anyway. Social support is critical to successful reintegration.
- Review BATTLEMIND to understand where some of your automatic behaviors come from.
- Remind your loved ones that you love them.
- Realize that you need to talk about the experiences you had during deployment. If you can't talk to family or friends, be sure to talk to a chaplain or counselor.

Red Flags

You now know the reactions that are normal following deployment to war. But sometimes the behaviors that kept you alive in the war zone get you on the wrong track at home. You may not be able to shut them down after you've returned home safely. Some problems may need outside assistance to solve.

Even serious post-deployment psychological problems can be treated successfully and cured. Being able to admit you have a problem can be tough:

- You might think you should cope on your own.
- You think others can't help you.

- You believe the problem(s) will go away on their own.
- You are embarrassed to talk to someone about it.

If your reactions are causing significant distress or interfering with how you function, you will need outside assistance. Things to watch for include

- Relationship troubles—frequent and intense conflicts, poor communication, inability to meet responsibilities
- Work, school, or other community dysfunction—frequent absences, conflicts, inability to meet deadlines or concentrate, poor performance
- Thoughts of hurting someone, or yourself

If you get assistance early, you can prevent more serious problems from developing. If you delay seeking help because of avoidance or stigma, your problems may actually cause you to lose your job, your relationships, and your happiness. Mental and emotional problems can be managed or treated, and early detection is essential.

Many of the common reactions to experience in a war zone are also symptoms of more serious problems such as PTSD. In PTSD, however, they're much more intense and troubling, and they don't go away. If these symptoms don't decrease over a few months, or if they continue to cause significant problems in your daily life, it's time to seek treatment from a professional.

COPING WITH TRAUMATIC STRESS REACTIONS
A NATIONAL CENTER FOR PTSD FACT SHEET
Pamela Swales, Ph.D.

Importance of Active Coping

When veterans take direct action to cope with their stress reactions and trauma-related problems, they put themselves in a position of power and start to be less helpless. Active coping means recognizing and accepting the impact of trauma on your life, and taking direct coping action to improve things. It means actively coping even when there is no crisis; coping is an attitude of mind and a habit that must be strengthened.

Understanding the Recovery Process

Knowing how recovery happens puts you in more control of the recovery process. Recovery is an ongoing daily gradual process. It doesn't happen through being suddenly "cured."

Some amount of continuing reactions is normal and reflects a normal body and mind. Healing doesn't mean forgetting traumatic war experiences or having no emotional pain when thinking about them. Healing may mean fewer symptoms and less disturbing symptoms, greater confidence in ability to cope with your memories and reactions, and improved ability to manage emotions.

Coping with Traumatic Stress Reactions: Ways that DON'T Help

- Using drugs and alcohol as ways to reduce anxiety or relax, stop thinking about war experiences, or go to sleep. Alcohol and drug use cause more problems than they cure.
- Keeping away from other people. Social isolation means loss of support, friendship, and closeness with others, and more time to worry or feel hopeless and alone.
- Dropping out of pleasurable or recreational activities. This leads to less opportunity to feel good and feel a sense of achievement.
- Using anger to control others. Anger helps keep other people away and may keep bad emotions away temporarily, but it also keeps away positive connections and help from loved ones.
- Trying to constantly avoid people, places, or thoughts that are reminders of the traumatic event. Avoidance of thinking about trauma or seeking treatment doesn't keep away distress, and it prevents progress on coping with stress reactions.
- Working all the time to try and avoid distressing memories of the trauma (the workaholic).

Coping with Traumatic Stress Reactions: Ways that CAN Help

There are many ways you can cope with post-traumatic stress. Here are some things you can do if you have any of the following symptoms:

Unwanted Distressing Memories, Images, or Thoughts

- Remind yourself that they are just that—memories.
- Remind yourself that it's natural to have some sorts of memories of the events(s).
- Talk to someone you trust about them.

- Remember that although reminders of trauma can feel overwhelming, they often lessen over time.

Sudden Feelings of Anxiety or Panic
- These are a common part of traumatic stress reactions, and include sensations of your heart pounding and feeling lightheaded or "spacey" (often due to rapid breathing). If this happens, remember that:
- These reactions are not dangerous. If you had them while exercising, they would not worry you.
- It is the addition of inaccurate frightening thoughts (e.g., I'm going to die, I'm having a heart attack, I will lose control) that makes them especially upsetting.
- Slowing down your breathing may help.
- The sensations will pass soon and you can still "go about your business" after they decrease.
- Each time you think in these positive ways about your arousal/anxious reactions, you will be helping them to happen less frequently. Practice will make it easier to cope.

Feeling Like the Trauma Is Happening Again (Flashbacks)
- Keep your eyes open. Look around you and notice where you are.
- Talk to yourself. Remind yourself where you are, what year you're in, and that you are safe.
- Trauma happened in the past, and you are in the present.
- Get up and move around. Have a drink of water, and wash your hands.
- Call someone you trust and tell them what's been happening.
- Remind yourself that this is a quite common traumatic stress reaction.
- Tell your counselor or doctor what happened to you.

Trauma-Related Dreams and Nightmares
- If you awaken from a nightmare in a "panic," remind yourself that you are reacting to a dream and that's why you are anxious/aroused . . . and not because there is real danger now.
- Consider getting up out of bed, "regrouping," and orienting yourself.
- Engage in a pleasant, calming activity (e.g., listen to soothing music).
- Talk to someone if possible.

- Talk to your doctor about your nightmares; certain medications can be helpful.

Difficulty Falling or Staying Asleep

- Keep to a regular bedtime schedule.
- Avoid strenuous exercise within a few hours of going to bed.
- Avoid using your sleeping area for anything other than sleeping or sexual intimacies.
- Avoid alcohol, tobacco, and caffeine. These harm your ability to sleep.
- Do not lie in bed thinking or worrying. Get up and enjoy something soothing or pleasant.
- Read a calming book, drink a glass of warm milk, do a quiet hobby.

Irritability, Anger, and Rage

- Take a "time-out" to cool off or to think things over. Walk away from the situation.
- Get in the habit of using daily exercise as a friend. Exercise reduces body tension and helps get the "anger out" in a positive and productive way.
- Remember that anger doesn't work. It actually increases your stress and can cause health problems.
- Talk to your counselor or doctor about your anger. Take classes in anger management.
- If you blow up at your family or friends, find time as soon as you are able to talk to them about it. Let them know how you feel, and what you are doing to cope with your reactions.

Difficulty Concentrating

- Slow down. Give yourself time to focus on what it is you need to learn or do.
- Write things down. Making to-do lists may be helpful.
- Break tasks down into small doable "chunks."
- Plan a realistic number of events or tasks for each day.
- Perhaps you may be depressed; many who are have trouble concentrating. Again, this is something you can discuss with your counselor, doctor, or someone close to you.

Having Difficulty Feeling or Expressing Positive Emotions

- Remember that this is a common reaction to trauma, that you are not doing this on purpose, and that you should not feel guilty for something you do not want to happen and cannot control.
- Make sure to regularly participate in activities that you enjoy or used to enjoy. Sometimes these activities can rekindle feelings of pleasure.
- Take steps to communicate caring to loved ones in little ways: write a card, leave a small gift, phone and say hello.

Experiment with these ways of coping to find which ones are helpful to you. Practice them, because, like other skills, they work better with practice. Talk to your counselor or doctor about them. Reach out to people in VA, Vet Centers, your family, and your community that can help. You're not alone.

*   *   *

SLEEP PROBLEMS
A NATIONAL CENTER FOR PTSD FACT SHEET

Julia M. Whealin, Ph.D.

Many people who have been deployed for combat or peacekeeping experience sleep problems, for various reasons. Some individuals may suffer from nightmares related to the deployment, and wake up feeling terrified. Others may feel the need to stay awake to protect themselves from danger. For example, some service members who have been in combat feel a need to "stand guard" at night, rather than sleep. Individuals may also have poor sleep habits that lead to insomnia, such as extended napping or an irregular sleep schedule.

What Can I Do If I Am Having Sleep Problems?

We are creatures of habit. Our sleep habits can either make sleeping easier or more difficult. The following ten suggestions have been shown to help reduce sleep problems:

1. Keep bed only for sleep—Do not watch TV, talk on the phone, review work, study, or solve problems while in bed. Go to bed only when you are drowsy and ready for sleep.
2. If you don't fall asleep within thirty minutes, get up—Go to another room and do something relaxing until you feel drowsy.

3. "Wind down" before bedtime—Do something calming, like light reading, listening to soothing music, praying, taking a warm bath, doing a crossword puzzle, or playing an enjoyable computer game before bedtime.

4. Have a regular bedtime and rising time—Go to sleep and wake up at the same time every day.

5. Limit naps—A midday nap as short as ten minutes can improve mood and mental performance. However, limit your nap to fifteen minutes and don't take it later than 4 p.m., or the nap may interfere with your sleep cycle.

6. Increase regular exercise—Just not too close to bedtime.

7. Decrease stimulants—Avoid smoking, or drinking coffee or soda with caffeine in the afternoon or evening.

8. Decrease alcohol—Because alcohol causes midnight awakenings, have no more than one serving of alcohol with dinner. Of course if you are in recovery from alcohol abuse, it is important to avoid alcohol entirely.

9. Inspect your bedroom environment—Is your bedroom dark and free of noise? Is your bed comfortable? Is the temperature comfortable? Do you feel safe and serene in your bedroom? If not, you can add images that are calming—a picture of your children, pet, an outdoor scene, a poem, or a prayer—to your room.

10. Get help—There are treatments that can help your sleep problems. If you continue to have sleep problems, see a trained sleep specialist to help identify what is the best treatment for you.

What If I Am Having Nightmares?

After a traumatic event, many people experience nightmares. For some, nightmares may continue to repeat for a long period of time. During nightmares, you may feel like you are "reliving" the event, with the same fear, helplessness, or rage experienced during the original trauma. Nightmares are not a sign that you are "going crazy." They are a way of working through a trauma.

Some people try to avoid nightmares by using drugs or alcohol, or by avoiding sleep altogether. These "solutions" only lead to new problems, such as substance dependence and sleep deprivation. When you wake up from a nightmare, leave the bedroom and go to another room to get your bearings. It may take a while to reorient yourself to the present. Do something relaxing. If possible, reach out to someone who supports you. If you live with others, discuss the fact that you are having nightmares. Discuss ways in which you might want to handle the situation and share this information with them. A small percentage of sufferers act out their nightmare in their sleep. You may want to rearrange your bedroom so that you are safe. If you share your bed with a partner, you may need to make sure he or she is not in harm's way.

How Are Sleep Problems Treated?

There are effective treatments for sleep problems. Choosing one that is right for you will depend on the situation. Medications are available for quick, short-term relief of insomnia and nightmares. Some medications can be addictive, however, so check with your doctor to find out which is best for you.

Some "talk therapies" will help bring about long-term relief of sleep problems. Cognitive-behavioral therapy targets your beliefs and behaviors that can make sleep problems worse. Sleep hygiene therapy helps people develop habits that can improve sleep. Breathing and relaxation therapies also may be used to help reduce muscle tension and promote sleep.

Therapies to treat nightmares are also available. For example, imagery rehearsal therapy focuses upon helping people change the endings of their nightmares, while they are awake, so the dream is no longer upsetting. This therapy has been shown to reduce nightmares in survivors of combat and sexual assault.

Where Can I Find More Information about Sleep Problems?

National Center for Post-Traumatic Stress Disorder: www.ptsd.va.gov/

National Alliance on Mental Illness: www.nami.org/Content/Content Groups/Helpline1/Sleep_Disorders.htm

Stanford University Center for Excellence in the Diagnosis and Treatment of Sleep Disorders: www.med.stanford.edu/school/psychiatry/coe/

Benefits

PAY AND ALLOWANCES

You may be concerned about how your pay and allowances will be impacted while you are recovering from a serious injury or illness. This section will give you a broad view of the most common pay questions recovering service members have.

Remember that your eligibility for pay is based on your personal situation, so if you have questions about pay, you should talk with your chain of command, your local pay office, or the Wounded Warrior Pay Management Team (WWPMT) representative where you are located. Some pay benefits are available only for those members who become injured or ill in combat-related circumstances. Others are available for anyone being treated for an illness or injury, or who is undergoing evaluation as part of the Disability Evaluation System (DES).

DISABILITY EVALUATION SYSTEM

When you become wounded, injured, or ill as a member of the armed forces, a formal set of rules is in place to make sure you receive all of the benefits for which you are eligible. This process is called the Disability Evaluation System (DES) and it operates under public law (Title 10 and Title 38) to ensure you are treated fairly.

Each military department has established its own procedures under public law and Department of Defense (DoD) guidelines for running the DES. While there are some differences among the services, all have the same general steps:

1. Evaluate service member's fitness for duty
2. Authorize a return to duty for those members who are found fit

3. Approve disability separations or retirements, to include making a benefits determination, for those service members who are found unfit

When you suffer a wound, illness, or injury, the doctors and staff of an
appropriate medical facility will treat you. For many members, this is the end
of the process if they are cured of the disease or fully recover from their
wound or injury. For a small number of members, a wound, illness, or injury
can result in a permanent condition that may make them unfit for continued
duty in their current job. If you suffer a permanent or long-lasting effect
from a wound, illness, or injury, the doctor will refer you to the DES process
by writing a narrative summary of your condition. The doctor sends your
case summary and a copy of your medical record to the nearest designated
military treatment facility commander, who assigns a Physical Evaluation
Board Liaison Officer (PEBLO) to assist you in your steps through the DES
process.

Each service uses a slightly different method to enter a member into the
DES. Additionally, because of unique missions and the individual member's
job classification, retention standards can vary. The Army, for instance, uses
a physical profile system that measures soldiers' physical limitations in six
areas with a level between 1 (fully healthy) to a 4 (severely limited) in each.
If a soldier receives a permanent level 3 or 4 in any area, the doctor is required to recommend that a Medical Evaluation Board (MEB) review the
soldier's case. The Air Force evaluates a member for retention and if his or
her condition(s) is limiting (not unfitting) they will assign an assignment
limitation code and reevaluate the member at a later date. If the condition is
not expected to improve within twelve months and the condition is permanently unfitting, they will be referred to an MEB. In the Navy and Marine
Corps, the process begins with the doctor writing the narrative summary and
no prior profiling requirement exists. You should talk with your chain of
command and your doctors to find out how the DES process begins for your
service.

The Medical Evaluation Board

Once you have been assigned a PEBLO, an MEB will review your record
to decide if you meet your service's medical retention standards. While each
service has individual rules, generally the MEB is made up of medical care
professionals, and in the case of mental health conditions, includes a mental

health care provider as well. The PEBLO will build a packet of information containing your medical records, results from tests and medical exams performed for the MEB related to your condition, letters from your chain of command related to how the injury or illness impacts your duty, copies of your performance evaluation reports, and other personnel records that the MEB may require. Every patient is different, and in some cases a doctor will wait to write the narrative summary until he or she sees how you respond to treatment and rehabilitation therapy before referring you to the MEB. The doctor will refer your case to the MEB only after he or she is satisfied that he or she has done all that can be medically done to improve your condition, though the services generally require doctors to initiate an MEB after a year of treatment for the same injury or illness.

When the MEB members review your case, they are responsible for answering the question "Do you meet the retention standards for your service?" In answering this question, there are several decisions they can make. They may determine that you meet medical retention standards and return you to full duty in your current job. They may determine that you meet medical retention standards in another job and recommend you retrain for that position. If they determine that you do not meet the medical retention standards, they will forward a recommendation to the Physical Evaluation Board (PEB).

Notice that the MEB does not determine your fitness for duty or level of disability.

The Physical Evaluation Board

The Department of Defense (DoD) regulations list minimum requirements for the membership of a PEB, but leaves the exact determination of who will sit on the boards up to the military department to decide. Generally, the services have opted for a three-person PEB, with a mix of military and civilian members. The president of the PEB is generally a colonel or a Navy captain, and the other board members include a field-grade personnel officer and a senior medical officer.

This ensures that each board has the expertise of a line officer in the president of the board, the medical knowledge of a senior medical officer, and the personnel policy knowledge of a senior personnel officer. The PEB will usually meet informally to review your case and will not require you to attend the informal meeting. Using the packet developed by the PEBLO during the MEB process, the board will review your medical record, the doctor's narrative summary, and your personnel evaluations and will determine if you are fit or unfit for continued service. The members will determine the severity of any disability you may have, with a rating between 0 and 100 percent using the VA Schedule for Rating Disabilities (VASRD). The members will then determine your disposition—return to duty, separation, or permanent or temporary retirement.

The PEBLO will notify you of the findings of the informal PEB. At this point, you have to choose between requesting a formal PEB or accepting the informal PEB findings. If you choose to have a formal PEB hearing, you will be allowed to appear before the PEB and discuss your case with the board members to ask them to reconsider their decision. You can also provide them additional information important to that reconsideration. Additionally, you have a right to be represented by legal counsel at the formal PEB.

The DES Pilot

Before 2007, all military members faced additional physical evaluations and disability ratings after leaving the military to receive benefits from the Department of Veterans Affairs (VA). While both the DoD and VA use the same rating tool, the VASRD, each had a different physical exam process. Additionally, they came to their own decision on percentages of disability to award as a result of the exam, sometimes leading to differences between VA and the DoD rating of the same injury or illness. The additional requirements led to delays in receiving VA benefits.

The President's Commission on Care for America's Returning Wounded Warriors, sometimes called the Dole-Shalala Report, recommended removing this dual-evaluation process and applying one medical exam and one rating determination by VA that the DoD could use for determining fitness at the PEB. In November 2007, the DoD and VA initiated a joint DES Pilot program in the National Capital Region (NCR) to improve the timelines, effectiveness, and transparency of the DES review process. The DoD and VA are evaluating the results of the pilot program and hope to expand the pilot's benefits to all recovering service members.

The pilot program allows military members to file a VA disability claim when they are referred to the DES. In the pilot program, the DoD relies on VA to perform the full medical exam used by the MEB and PEB to determine if the member meets service retention standards and, later, by the PEB to determine if the member is fit to remain in the service. VA provides a disability rating for each condition found during the medical exam, and the PEB uses these ratings to determine the type of separation or retirement for which the member is eligible.

Although the DoD and VA expect the pilot program to be faster and fairer, you should understand that, even in the pilot program, there are still differences in the final, combined DoD and VA disability percentage. The DoD, by law, can only consider conditions that are unfitting when determining disability ratings, while VA determines disability ratings for all service-connected conditions, even the ones that would not result in a finding of unfit for continued military service. The DoD uses the VA disability percentages for each condition, but may have a different combined disability rating than VA awards because conditions that are not unfitting are not considered in the DoD calculations.

Understanding Disability Ratings and Benefits

If the PEB finds you unfit based on one or more of your conditions, they will provide you with a combined disability ratings percentage. This is an important number because it determines what type of separation you receive and, subsequently, the types of benefits you are eligible to receive from the DoD. VA benefits are also discussed in chapter 7 of this guide.

Some veterans are confused when they receive a higher, combined disability rating from VA than from the DoD. It is important for you to remember that the PEB calculates your combined rating based only on conditions that make you unfit for continued service. So, if the VA finds that you have disabilities that are connected to your military service but that did not make you unfit for service, you will receive a higher disability rating from the VA than from the DoD. This difference is required by law and applies even if you are taking part in the DES Pilot program and receive your medical examination and disability evaluation from VA.

The combined disability rating is not calculated by adding the percentage of disability for each condition rated "unfitting." Rather, the highest disability rating is considered first, then the next highest, and so on in order of severity. If you have a 60 percent disability, the VA Schedule for Rating Disabilities (VASRD) considers you to be 40 percent "efficient." Efficiency is the measure of your total health minus your disability, so someone with a 60 percent disability has only 40 percent of his or her total health that is not impacted by the disability. The next highest disability percentage will be applied to the 40 percent efficiency left after the initial 60 percent rating is applied to the total healthy score of 100 percent efficient.

The following example involves a member with three unfitting conditions rated 60, 30, and 20 percent:

- First rating is 60 percent of the whole person, leaving the member with 40 percent efficiency.
- Second rating is 30 percent of the 40 percent efficiency, which is a loss of 12 percent efficiency (.30 x .40 = .12). This is added to the original disability percentage of 60, for a cumulative score of 72 percent combined disability from the first two conditions. This leaves the member with 28 percent efficiency.
- Third rating is 20 percent of the 28 percent efficiency, which is a loss of 6 percent efficiency (.20 x .28 = 5.6, which is rounded up to 6). Added to the combined disability in the second rating of 72, the rating becomes 78 percent.
- The combined rating of 78 percent must be rounded to the nearest 10, giving the member a combined rating of 80 percent.

The math can be complicated. The VASRD uses a table in Section 4.25 (table 1) of Title 38 of the Code of Federal Regulations (CFR) to allow you to determine your combined rating if you would like to do so, but the rating will be combined for you by the PEB and VA for use in determining benefits they will provide to you. You can find a copy of the sections of Title 38 related to combined ratings online by going to www.access.gpo.gov/nara/cfr/waisidx_04/38cfr4_04.html and scrolling down to Section 4.25.

PEB Disposition Finding

When the PEB provides its final disposition of your case, there are five possible outcomes. These outcomes are based on your combined rating, based on the "unfitting" conditions. The dispositions available from the PEB are

- Return to duty: If your conditions are not considered severe enough to make you unfit for duty, you will be returned to your job and service. No disability benefits are required, since you are allowed to continue in the service, though when you someday separate from the military, you may be eligible for benefits from the VA for a service-connected disability that could impact your earning potential after you leave the military.

- Separate with severance pay: If one or more of your conditions is considered unfitting for continued service in the military, but the combined disability of all your unfitting conditions is between 0 and 20 percent, you may receive severance pay based on your time in service and current pay grade. The local finance office, or the Defense Finance and Accounting Service (DFAS) Wounded Warrior Pay Management Team (WWPMT), will help you calculate the amount of severance pay you are authorized. However, if you have served at least twenty years and are eligible for retirement, you will instead be retired from service as explained below.

- Separate without benefits: Some injuries are determined to be "not in the line of duty." These are injuries that are a result of intentional misconduct or willful negligence on your part or that took place when you were not on orders if you are a National Guard or Reserve member. If your injury is found to be not in the line of duty but is unfitting, you could be separated without benefits for those injuries. If your injury or illness resulted from a medical problem that you had before you entered service, and the injury or illness was not aggravated by your service, you may also be separated without benefits. There are some special rules for this situation. If you have served more than six months in the military, you could be eligible for benefits unless there is compelling medical evidence showing that the condition existed at the same level of severity before you joined. Your PEBLO can help you understand the rules for separation without disability benefits.

- Permanent Disability Retirement List (PDRL): If all your unfitting conditions result in a combined disability rating of 30 percent or higher, and your condition is considered stable (meaning it is unlikely, in the doctor's opinion, that your disability rating will change within five years), you will be permanently retired for disability and placed on the PDRL. This provides you with disability retirement pay, access to TRICARE for you and your dependent family members enrolled in the Defense Enrollment Eligibility Reporting System (DEERS), access to commissary and exchange shopping, and all other benefits of regular military retirement. If you have more than twenty years in service, and your combined disability rating is 0 to 20 percent, you will be allowed to retire with all the regular retirement benefits. The local finance office or the DFAS Wounded Warrior Pay Management Team will help you calculate the amount of retirement pay you will receive.

- Temporary Disability Retirement List (TDRL): The TDRL allows the service to ensure a medical condition stabilizes before making a final disability determination. If you are eligible for permanent disability retirement, but your condition is not considered stable, you will be temporarily retired and placed on the TDRL for a maximum of five years. Every twelve to eighteen months, you will be reevaluated to see if your condition has stabilized and if you can reenter the service. The benefits of the TDRL are the same as those you would have received had you been retired under the PDRL. If, during those five years, the service determines that your condition is stable and you are fit for duty, your service will offer you the chance to return to duty. If your condition stabilizes but you are not able to return to duty, you will be permanently retired.

How to Appeal Decisions of the PEB for Your Service

Army

Your case will go before the informal PEB without you being present. Only your record from the MEB will go to this board. The PEB will discuss your case and return a disposition.

If you are found fit, you can either concur (agree) or non-concur (disagree) with the board's findings. If you non-concur, you will be allowed to present a written rebuttal to the PEB regarding why you disagree. This is your chance to provide more information on your condition and how it affects your duty performance. Because you were found fit, you do not have a right to a formal PEB where you can discuss your case in person. However, you can request a formal PEB as an exception to policy.

If you are found unfit, you can agree or disagree with the findings. Like the appeal of a fit decision, you may send a written rebuttal to the PEB with new information on your condition and its effects on your duty performance. However, because you were found unfit, you also have the right to a formal hearing and, if you would like, you may appear at the hearing in person.

You may seek legal assistance to prepare for a formal PEB. You may be represented at the hearing by an attorney from the Judge Advocate General (JAG) Corps, or you can choose a civilian attorney or a representative from a Veterans Service Organization (VSO), like the Disabled American Veterans. If you choose to use your own counsel and not a representative from the JAG Corps, you will be responsible for any fees or payments that come from bringing in an outside counsel. Legal representation from the JAG Corps is free to you.

When you appear before a formal PEB, you may present evidence, testimony, and documents to support your case. Your legal representative will help you prepare for this.

The formal PEB will listen to your new information, ask you questions about your medical limitations, and give you a chance to make a final statement before they make a decision. You will be excused from the hearing after your statement, and the PEB members will discuss and vote on your case. The formal PEB makes decisions by majority vote. If some members of the board disagree with the majority, they must write a minority opinion that will become part of the report of proceedings that documents the board's actions.

The board will bring you and your counsel back into the room and tell you their decision. They will also provide you a written copy of the report of proceedings. You will have ten calendar days after the board ends to decide if you agree or disagree with its findings.

If you disagree, you will again have an opportunity to provide a written rebuttal to the formal PEB. If the PEB does not accept your rebuttal and upholds its decision, your case will go to the U.S. Army Physical Disability Agency (USAPDA) for review. All cases decided by informal or formal PEBs are sent to the USAPDA, but only those where the soldier disagrees with the findings or where there is a minority report written are automatically reviewed. The USAPDA also reviews about 20 percent of the rest of the cases to spot-check PEB consistency and accuracy.

The USAPDA can uphold the PEB findings, issue revised findings, or send the case back to the PEB for another review. If the USAPDA revises the findings or sends the case back to the PEB for another review, you will again have the chance to agree or disagree with the findings and to provide a written rebuttal to the PEB before the findings are completed. If you didn't request a formal review before, you may request one based on revised findings by the USAPDA, and the formal review will take place at that level. Once the USAPDA makes a final decision on your case, you will have to follow that disposition. If that requires separation or retirement, then you will be separated or retired. However, you may still dispute the findings after you have separated or retired by filing a petition for relief with the Army Board for the Correction of Military Records (ABCMR) if you believe the findings are incorrect.

You can find out more about your appeal rights by reviewing the *Army Physical Disabilities Evaluation System Handbook*, dated March 16, 2007. You can find a copy of that handbook by visiting the website www.cs.amedd. army.mil/apdes/docs/General%20and%20Reference%20Information/Army_ PDES_booklet.doc.

Navy/Marine Corps

The Navy and Marine Corps use the same PEB process. Like the other services, this process begins with an informal PEB and only moves to a formal PEB if the sailor or marine requests it.

The informal PEB will take place without you being present, and the board will decide your disposition based on your records and the MEB results. If the board finds you fit for duty, you will have an opportunity to agree or disagree with that decision. You can write a request for reconsideration to the board with new information on your medical condition and any other information the board did not have when reviewing your record. You also need to tell the board if you would like a formal PEB if they uphold the fit decision. Keep in mind that a formal PEB is not a right if you are found fit for continued naval service, and the board may choose not to grant you a formal PEB.

If you are found unfit, you have three choices. You can accept the findings of the PEB, disagree with the finding and request a formal PEB, or conditionally accept the findings and request a formal PEB.

If you request a formal PEB, the Navy will assign a judge advocate to help you prepare evidence, documents, and statements to support your case. You may attend the formal PEB in person or just send information to the board. You may also choose to be represented by a civilian attorney of your choice or a representative from a Veterans Service Organization (VSO), but you will be responsible for any costs that arise from using a nonmilitary appointed lawyer. If you choose not to testify under oath, you will be allowed to make a statement, but the board members will not ask you questions. If you choose to testify under oath, the board will ask you questions about your condition and the effect it has on your duty performance. After you have answered the board's questions, they will give you a chance to make a final statement then you will be excused while they make a decision on your case.

The board will tell you what it decided after they complete discussions of your case. At this point, you can either accept their findings, or you can file a petition for relief (PFR) with the Director, Secretary of the Navy Council of Review Boards (DIRSECNAVCORB). A PFR is another way to challenge the board's decision. The DIRSECNAVCORB can modify the findings of the board or uphold them.

If you are separated or retired and still disagree with the findings of the PEB or the DIRSECNAVCORB, you can petition the Board for Correction of Naval Records (BCNR) for relief from any perceived injustice or inequity.

For information on your rights before the formal PEB, visit the Navy legal webpage at www.donhq.navy.mil/corb/peb/?pebmainpage1.htm for more information.

Air Force

Like the other services, the Air Force PEB will start with an informal board that you do not attend. Your record will be forwarded from the MEB, and the informal PEB members will review it and decide your disposition. Within a few days of the board, your PEBLO will contact you to give you the results of the informal PEB. You will be asked to sign an Air Force Form 1180 to tell the PEB if you agree with the findings or not.

If you disagree with a finding of fit, you will need to write a justification for why you would like a formal PEB and submit that justification with the Air Force Form 1180. Like the other services, formal PEBs are not guaranteed when you receive a fit for continued duty finding.

If you are found unfit, you do not have to provide a justification for requesting a formal PEB. You will need to contact the legal office at Lackland Air Force Base, where the formal PEBs are held.

You can contact them at DSN 473-4295 or commercial 210-671-4295 to have a lawyer assigned to your case. You can also choose a civilian attorney or a representative from a VSO like the Disabled American Veterans. If you choose to use your own counsel and not a military lawyer, you will be responsible for any fees or payments that come from bringing in outside counsel. Legal representation from the military is free to you. When you appear before a formal PEB, you may present evidence, testimony, and documents to support your case. Your legal representative will help you prepare for this.

If you have witnesses you wish to testify in person, you will have to pay for the expense of bringing them to the formal PEB location. If, after meeting with your legal counsel, you decide that you do not want to do a formal PEB after all, you can waive your rights to a board. However, the president of the board will decide whether or not to hold a formal PEB once you have requested one. Audio of the formal PEB is recorded in all cases. If you request it, video of the proceedings can also be recorded.

After you have presented your information to the formal PEB, they will meet privately to make a decision on your case. The formal PEB will either uphold the informal PEB findings or recommend different findings. The board will notify you of their decision, and you will have a day to tell them if you agree or disagree with their findings.

If you agree with the formal PEB findings, your case will be sent to the Physical Disability Division at Headquarters, Air Force Personnel Command, for finalization. The Physical Disability Division will review your case, the findings of the informal and formal PEB, and decide if your case should be finalized or forwarded for further review by the Secretary of the Air Force Personnel Council (SAFPC). This only happens when the Physical Disability Division thinks a review by the SAFPC is in your best interest or the best interest of the Air Force.

If you disagree with the formal PEB findings, you will have ten days to submit a rebuttal to the formal PEB for forwarding to the SAFPC. If the formal PEB does not receive your rebuttal in that time, your case will go to the Physical Disability Division for processing.

Even if the SAFPC upholds the formal PEB and you are separated or retired, you may still appeal that decision by applying to the Air Force Board for Correction of Military Records (AFBCMR). This is the highest administrative appeal available for the Air Force. The burden of proof is on you to show that an error or injustice happened in your case during the DES process.

You can get additional information on the Air Force appeals process at http://airforcemedicine.afms.mil/idc/groups/public/documents/webcontent/ knowledgejunction.hcst?functionalarea = LeadersGuideDistress&doctype = subpage&docname = CTB_030792

PHYSICAL DISABILITY EVALUATION SYSTEM

There are different dispositions the PEB can determine for your service unfitting conditions. Three of those dispositions—discharge with severance,

TDRL, and PDRL—will result in you receiving compensation from the government. You should contact your local finance or personnel office, or the WWPMT member at your location, to get details about your particular situation.

Severance Pay

For those who receive a severance pay rather than disability retirement, the pay is calculated by taking your base pay, multiplying it by two, and multiplying that number by the number of years of service you have completed. The minimum multiplier for years of service, regardless of the number of years you have served, will be three years of service or, for those injured in a combat zone, six years of service. So, if you are separated after only two years' service, you will receive credit for three years of service when calculating your severance or six years if you were injured in a combat zone. Because those with twenty or more years of service are given retirement pay regardless of their combined disability rating, the maximum severance multiplier for years of service is nineteen.

Severance Pay Calculation Example

The calculation for an E-4 with two years of service in 2008 separated for a non-combat-zone injury would be

$$\$1,848.90 \text{ (base pay)} \times 2 = \$3,697.80$$
$$\$3,697.80 \times 3 \text{ (minimum number of years service for non-combat-zone injury)} = \$11,093.40 \text{ lump sum}$$

For the same E-4 with two years of service in 2008, but who was injured in a combat zone, the calculation would be

$$\$1,848.90 \text{ (base pay)} \times 2 = \$3,697.80$$
$$\$3,697.80 \times 6 \text{ (minimum years service for combat-zone injury)} = \$22,186.80$$

Temporary Disability Retirement List (TDRL)

If the PEB finds you unfit for duty with a 30 percent or higher combined disability rating, but your condition is not considered stable (it may worsen or improve), then you will be placed on the TDRL. Your compensation under TDRL is determined using one of two methods based on Formula

Number 2 found in United States Code (U.S.C.), Title 10, Chapter 71, Section 1401.

Under the first method, your retirement is based on your combined disability percentage, but can never be less than 50 percent of your current base pay. Additionally, retirement pay can never be more than 75 percent of base pay, so a combined rating of 80–100 percent will result in retirement compensation equal to 75 percent base pay.

- 30–40 percent disability rating = 50 percent of base pay
- 50–70 percent disability rating = that percentage of base pay
- 80–100 percent disability rating = 75 percent of base pay
- or 2.5 percent x years of service if sum is greater than percentage of disability

Under the second method, your retirement is based on your time in service using the formulas in U.S.C., Title 10, Chapter 71, Section 1401 (http://uscode.house.gov/download/title_10.shtml).

Under this method, your compensation would be determined by taking 2.5 percent multiplied by the total number of years' service you have to come up with the percentage of retired pay.

- 2.5 percent x years of service = that percentage of base pay

Your TDRL payment will be based on the method that gives you the highest percentage of base pay. You will never be placed on the TDRL with less than 50 percent of base pay.

Every eighteen months, you will have a physical exam to see if your condition has changed or if it has stabilized. Those examinations will determine whether you remain on TDRL, return to duty, are discharged with or without severance, or are moved to the PDRL.

- If you are fit for duty, you will have the choice of returning to duty or being discharged without severance. Your TDRL payments will stop.
- If your condition has stabilized, and you are still unfit for duty with a disability between 0 and 20 percent, you will be discharged with severance.
- If your condition has stabilized and your disability is rated at 30 percent or higher, you will be transferred to the PDRL.

At the end of five years, you must be declared fit or unfit, given a percentage of disability, and either returned to duty, discharged, or placed on PDRL.

Permanent Disability Retired List (PDRL)

If you are found unfit by the PEB with a 30 percent or greater combined disability rating, and your condition is considered stable (unlikely to improve), you will be placed on the PDRL. You will also be placed on PDRL if you have less than 30 percent disability, but have completed twenty or more years of service.

Your retired pay will be determined using Formula Number 1 of United States Code, Title 10, Chapter 71, Section 1401. It is much like the method used to determine TDRL retired pay but without the 50 percent minimum. In other words, you will receive retirement pay based on your combined disability rating percentage, or you will receive retirement pay based on your years of service. Like TDRL, you receive the amount that is greater of the two methods for determining the pay, but it cannot exceed 75 percent of base pay.

- 30–70 percent disability rating = that percentage of base pay
- 80–100 percent disability rating = 75 percent of base pay
- or 2.5 percent x years of service if sum is greater than percentage of disability

Combat-Related Special Compensation (CRSC)

Historically, veterans have not been allowed to receive both military retirement pay and disability compensation from VA. Effective June 1, 2003, a law allowed retired members with twenty years' service and qualifying combat-related disabilities to receive special payments that lessened the offset of VA compensation for combat-related disabilities that reduced DoD retirement payments. This law was expanded by the 2008 National Defense Authorization Act (NDAA) to include members who are retired with less than twenty years for medical reasons. Eligible veterans with VA-rated disabilities that have been determined to be combat-related and who have twenty or more years of creditable service, who are permanent medical retirees, or who have been placed on the TDRL, are eligible for a monthly CRSC payment in addition to their reduced military retirement pay and their VA disability compensation. Each service uses a different process for determining eligibility. Talk to your chain of command about your situation, or contact your service CRSC experts at the following address:

Department of the Army
Combat-Related Special Compensation (CRSC)
200 Stovall Street
Alexandria, VA 22332-0470
Phone: 866-281-3254
Website: www.crsc.army.mil

Air Force
United States Air Force
Disability Division (CRSC)
550 C Street West Ste 6
Randolph AFB TX 78150-4708
Phone: 800-616-3775
Website: www.afpc.randolph.af.mil/library/combat.asp

Coast Guard
Commander (adm-1-CRSC)
U.S. Coast Guard
Personnel Command
4200 Wilson Boulevard
Arlington, VA 22203-1804
Website: www.uscg.mil/hr/psc

Navy and Marine Corps
Secretary of the Navy Council of Review Boards
Attn: Combat-Related Special Compensation Board
720 Kennon Street SE, Suite 309
Washington Navy Yard, DC 20374
Phone: 877-366-2772
Website: www.hq.navy.mil/corb/CRSCB/combatrelated.htm

Concurrent Retirement and Disability Payments (CRDP)

Another program designed to remove the offset of VA and DoD payments is the CRDP. The CRDP program provides a ten-year phase-out of the offset to military retired pay from receiving VA disability compensation for members who have a combined disability rating of 50 percent or greater. Members retired under disability provisions must have twenty years of service. See your chain of command or VA advisor to discuss how to apply for CRDP.

Access to Special/Partial/Casual Pays

If you are being treated at a location that makes it difficult for you to get to your bank, you may be eligible for a special payment to cover incidental costs that come up during your treatment. The Army calls these "casual pays," the Air Force calls them "partial pays," and the Navy/Marine Corps call them "special pays." This is an advance on your end-of-month paycheck and will be automatically deducted from pay during subsequent pay periods until paid back. The finance office closest to where you are located can help you with this request.

Basic Allowance for Subsistence (BAS)

If you are hospitalized, you will continue to receive your BAS while you are an inpatient. When you are an outpatient, you will continue to receive BAS as long as you are not issued a meal card to eat in the military dining facility. Contact your chain of command or administrative support section to determine your specific eligibility.

PAY ISSUES SPECIFIC TO COMBAT ZONE INJURIES/ILLNESSES

Pay and Allowance Continuation (PAC)

If you are hospitalized for treatment from a wound, illness, or injury you received in a combat zone, hostile fire area, or from being exposed to a hostile fire event, you continue to receive all pay and allowances (including any bonus, incentive pay, or similar benefit) that you were getting when you were wounded, injured, or became ill. PAC continues for up to one year after you are first hospitalized. The Principal Under Secretary of Defense for Personnel and Readiness can extend PAC beyond the one-year limit for six-month periods under "extraordinary circumstances" under the authority of U.S.C., Title 37, Section 372.

You should discuss your situation with your WWPMT contact or the chain of command to find out if you are eligible for PAC.

Filing a Travel Voucher for Your Time in a Combat Zone

If you are evacuated from a combat zone for medical treatment, you will receive per diem for the day you travel to and from that area. You are also allowed to claim $3.50 in incidental expenses for each day you were deployed to a combat zone. To receive this money, you will need to file a travel voucher (DD Form 1351-2).

If you are being treated as an inpatient at a medical facility, you are not eligible for travel pay on those dates. When you are treated as an outpatient at a medical facility, you may also be eligible for travel pay, depending on where you are being treated. Each service handles travel payments differently. The Army travel pay is handled by the DFAS Casualty Travel, Indianapolis office.

The Navy, Air Force, and Marine Corps handle the travel pay at their local finance offices. If you have questions, you should contact your nearest finance office and ask for the WWPMT point of contact. More information is also available by going to www.dfas.mil/travelpay.html and choosing the information for your service.

Travel for Your Family

Your family may want to be with you during your treatment to support you in your recovery. If you are being treated at a location away from your family, they may be able to travel at government expense to be with you. Travel for your family is handled much like other military travel and requires submitting a travel voucher for payment. The orders for your family will be called Invitational Travel Authorizations (ITAs), Invitational Travel Orders (ITOs), or Emergency Family Member Travel (EFMT) orders, depending upon your service. Up to three members of your immediate family may be eligible to travel to your location while you are an inpatient. When you become an outpatient, the local finance office can provide one family member orders to remain with you during your recovery. Family members who are eligible for this travel include parents, spouses, children, or siblings. Like your travel orders, incremental payments and extensions to the orders may be needed if your stay as an inpatient or outpatient at the medical facility is an extended one. The ITAs/ITOs/EFMTs will cover the cost of travel, hotel bills, meals, and some incidentals up to a maximum daily amount determined by your location. Some expenses, like rental car costs, are not reimbursable. Each service handles the process of getting your family the orders and the reimbursement for costs in a slightly different manner.

- Army: The WWPMT at the local finance office will help your family fill out the travel vouchers needed to pay expenses. Additionally, your Army

Wounded Warrior (AW2) program advocate can help you get the process started. You can also get information from the DFAS Travel Pay customer service center by calling toll-free at 888-332-7366.

- Navy: The local Personnel Support Detachment (PSD) at the medical facility or installation will help your family fill out the travel vouchers and answer any questions about the maximum amount authorized for the location. Additionally, your Safe Harbor program advocate can help you get your family to your bedside. Navy families can also get additional information from the DFAS Travel Pay customer service center by calling toll-free 888-332-7366.

- Marine Corps: The Patient Administration Team (PAT) or the Inspector-Instructor (I-I) will give your family members their ITOs and can explain the maximum amounts of per diem at your location.

  The PAT and I-I will also provide extensions for the orders if needed, help with filing travel vouchers every thirty days to receive payment, help fill out requests for advances, and answer any questions your family members may have. You can call the Marine Corps Casualty Branch at 800-847-1597 or 703-784-9512. If calling over the DSN, the prefix is 278.

- Air Force: The Air Force appoints a Family Liaison Officer (FLO) for each Air Force member who suffers a combat-related wound, illness, or injury. The FLO will provide your family with the EFMT paperwork needed to get them to your location and will answer questions they may have. If you or your family have any unresolved issues or need more information on EFMT, call toll-free at 800-433-0048. The commercial number is 210-565-3505.

Family Separation Allowance (FSA)

This is a pay you receive if you have dependents and are away from your permanent duty station for more than thirty days for temporary duty or on a temporary change of station. If you were receiving FSA while deployed, then are sent to a medical facility for treatment in a location other than your permanent duty station, you will continue to be paid FSA unless all your dependents come to stay at your location for more than thirty days. The pay stops on the thirty-first day all your dependents are in your location. The pay stops on the day before you return to your permanent duty location. Contact the local pay office, or the WWPMT contact at your location for more information.

Hardship Duty Pay Location (HDP-L)

HDP-L is paid while you are in a location that the secretary of defense identifies as a hardship duty location. This entitlement stops on the day you leave the hardship location, unless you are covered by PAC (see above for an explanation of PAC).

Hostile Fire Pay/Imminent Danger Pay (HFP/IDP)

HFP/IDP is paid when you are in an area the president identifies as placing you in imminent danger or where you may come under hostile fire. Talk to someone at your pay office to learn what your monthly amount should be. You can also read DoD 7100.14-R, Vol. 7A, Ch. 10, Sect. 100102 or visit the DFAS website (www.dfas.mil). If you became wounded, injured, or ill while receiving HFP/IDP, you will continue receiving this pay while you are covered by PAC.

Combat Zone Tax Exclusion (CZTE)

If you were serving in a combat zone that provided CZTE benefits before you were medically evacuated, you will not be required to begin paying taxes for any month in which you are an inpatient being treated for wounds, illnesses, or injuries you received in that combat zone for up to two years after discharge or after the official end of hostilities.

If you are treated as an outpatient, your tax exclusion ends at the end of the month in which you were either transferred out of theater or moved from inpatient to outpatient status. If you are readmitted as an inpatient for treatment of the same injury or illness, you will receive tax exclusion for the month in which you are readmitted and for every month thereafter until you are discharged or the two-year period ends. Contact the WWPMT or local pay office to learn more about your particular situation.

Combat-Related Injury and Rehabilitation Pay (CIP)

The PAC program replaced CIP on May 15, 2008. Wounded Warriors are still eligible to claim retroactive periods of CIP qualification. CIP was an entitlement payable monthly. If you were medically evacuated out of a combat zone and considered "hospitalized," you were entitled to CIP. For the purposes of CIP entitlement, you were considered hospitalized if you were admitted as an inpatient or were receiving extensive rehabilitation as an outpatient while living in quarters affiliated with the military health care system.

An example of government affiliated quarters is the Fisher House at Walter Reed Army Medical Center. Entitlement to CIP ended upon receipt of TSGLI. Contact your local finance office if you believe you should have earned CIP but did not receive the entitlement.

Savings Deposit Program (SDP)

When you are deployed to an area that makes you eligible for HFP/IDP and are there for at least thirty consecutive days (or at least one day in three consecutive months), you are allowed to deposit up to $10,000 in a DoD savings account that receives a 10 percent interest rate. If you are evacuated, you may withdraw that money from your SDP account should you need the funds for immediate expenses. If you don't wish to withdraw right away, the DFAS will automatically transfer the balance of your SDP into your regular military pay 120 days after you leave the combat zone. If you wish to withdraw your money right away, you can fill out a withdrawal request form on the myPay website at mypay.dfas.mil/mypay.aspx. You can also withdraw your money by sending an e-mail to CCL-SDP@dfas.mil, or by sending a fax to 216-522-5060. You may also mail your request to

DFAS-Cleveland Center (DFAS-CL)
ATTN: SDP
Special Claims
1240 East 9th Street
Cleveland, OH 44199-2055

Your request for withdrawal must include your name, social security number, and the date you left the combat zone. Keep in mind that your SDP will continue to accrue interest for ninety days after you leave the combat zone, so withdrawal before that point will reduce the interest you receive on your savings. For more information, contact the SDP Help Line toll-free at 888-332-7411, commercial: 216-522-5096, or DSN: 580-5096. You can also request information via e-mail at CCL-SDP@dfas.mil.

Traumatic Servicemembers' Group Life Insurance (TSGLI)

Certain types of injuries that result in a severe loss, such as a leg or arm amputation, may entitle you to TSGLI payments. A more detailed explanation of eligibility and amounts is available in chapter 7.

You can call the SGLI office toll-free at 800-419-1473 or you can visit the TSGLI webpage at www.insurance.va.gov/sgliSite/TSGLI/TSGLI.htm for more information.

FAMILY AND MEDICAL LEAVE ACT

Members of your family may want to be with you while you are treated for an illness or injury. In the past, this meant some family members had to choose between employment and providing care for a service member.

The National Defense Authorization Act for Fiscal Year 2008 (Public Law 110-181) added protection for families of military members under the Family and Medical Leave Act. This means your family may have job protection when they take time off of work to care for you.

With the changes in the law, your family member may be eligible for up to twenty-six weeks of unpaid leave in a one-year period to care for you. For this benefit, you must have a serious injury or illness that occurred in the line of duty while on active duty.

Not all family members are eligible. Spouses, children, parents, and/or a next of kin are usually covered if they meet the requirements in the law for time worked at the place of employment. Other family members may be eligible in some cases.

Some employers are exempt from the law. For example, a business with less than fifty workers may be exempt.

The Department of Labor (DOL) offers your family members several ways to get information on eligibility. DOL has a webpage to explain who can use the Family and Medical Leave Act (FMLA), which can be found at www.dol.gov/whd/fmla/index.htm. If your family member feels he or she is eligible for unpaid leave under this law, but his or her employer disagrees, you can contact the DOL Wage and Hour Division. The division operates a toll-free hotline at 866-4US-WAGE (487-9243), which is operated from 8 a.m. to 8 p.m. Eastern time, Monday through Friday. This is a general information hotline that will refer you to the local DOL office for assistance. Local DOL offices are also listed on the DOL webpage at www.dol.gov/dol/location.htm.

DEPARTMENT OF VETERANS AFFAIRS BENEFITS

VA offers a host of programs that you may be eligible for, depending on your situation. To determine eligibility, you will need to file claims with VA. The

VA representative at your installation, or a VSO advisor, can help you with this process.

Compensation and Pension (VA Form 21-526)

You can file a VA claim for

- Disability compensation for a service-connected injury, continuing illness, mental or physical impairment, and/or permanent and combined disability
- Pension benefit if you served during a wartime period, have limited income, and have a non-service-connected permanent and combined disability

Disability compensation is a monthly payment to you if you are disabled by an injury or illness that was incurred or aggravated during active military service. How much you receive depends on the degree of disability and the number of dependents you have. Veterans with certain severe disabilities may be eligible for additional special monthly compensation. You do not pay federal or state income tax on disability compensation. The payment of military retirement pay, disability severance pay, and separation incentive payments known as SSB (Special Separation Benefits) and VSI (Voluntary Separation Incentives) affects the amount of VA compensation you may receive.

CRDP will restore your retired pay on a graduated ten-year schedule if you have a 50 to 90 percent VA-rated disability. Concurrent retirement payments increase 10 percent per year through 2013. If you are rated at 100 percent disabled by VA, you are entitled to full CRDP now.

CRSC provides tax-free monthly payments to eligible retired veterans with combat-related injuries. With CRSC, you are eligible for a monthly CRSC payment in addition to your reduced military retirement pay and VA disability compensation, with VA-rated, combat-related disabilities.

Increased Compensation Based on Unemployability (VA Form 21-8940)

This form is for compensation based on your unemployability due to total disability from service-connected disability(s) that prevent you from having a substantial occupation.

SGLI Disability Extension (SGLV 8715)

This form is used to apply for an extension of your SGLI coverage for two years from your date of discharge from the military at no cost if you are totally disabled. SGLI is a low-cost life insurance program for military members. You can find more information about the SGLI Disability Extension by going to www.insurance.va.gov or by calling the Office of Servicemembers' Group Life Insurance toll-free at 800-419-1473, Eastern time.

Servicemembers' Group Life Insurance Traumatic Injury Protection Payment (GL-2005.261)

This form helps you to receive insurance payment if you have service-connected traumatic injury or loss from your time during OEF/OIF.

Veterans' Group Life Insurance (VGLI) (SGLV 8714)

SGLI may be converted to VGLI, which provides renewable term coverage to

- Veterans who had full-time SGLI coverage upon release from active duty or the Reserves
- Ready Reservists with part-time SGLI coverage who incur a disability or aggravate a preexisting disability during a Reserve period that renders them uninsurable at standard premium rates
- Members of the Individual Ready Reserve and Inactive National Guard

SGLI can be converted to VGLI up to the amount of coverage you had when separated from service. If you submit an application and the initial premium within 120 days of leaving the service, you will be covered regardless of your health. After 120 days, you have an additional year to convert to VGLI if you submit an application, pay the initial premium, and show evidence of insurability within one year of termination of SGLI coverage. If you are totally disabled at the time of separation, you are eligible for the SGLI Disability Extension, which will provide SGLI at no cost for up to two years. Your SGLI Disability Extension is automatically converted to VGLI at the end of the extension period. VGLI is convertible at any time to a permanent plan policy with any participating commercial insurance company. SGLV 8714 is used to convert your SGLI to VGLI. For more information about VGLI, visit www.insurance.va.gov or call the Office of Servicemembers' Group Life Insurance toll-free at 800-419-1473.

Service-Disabled Veterans Insurance (VA Form 29-4364)

The Service-Disabled Veterans Insurance (S-DVI) program is a life insurance program designed to meet the insurance needs of certain veterans with service-connected disabilities. S-DVI is available in a variety of permanent plans as well as term insurance. Policies are issued for a maximum face amount of $10,000. In order to be eligible for S-DVI, you must have

- Received other than a dishonorable discharge
- Been released from active duty after April 25, 1951
- Received a rating for a new service-connected disability (even 0 percent) within the last two years

Note: The granting of individual unemployability or an increase for a previously rated condition does not provide a new eligibility period for S-DVI.

You must apply within two years from the date VA notifies you of your new service-connected disability. There are two ways you can apply for basic S-DVI:

1. Apply online using the AutoForm application.
   The web-based application will walk you through the application, step-by-step, and can be submitted electronically. The application can be accessed at www.insurance.va.gov/autoform/index.asp.
2. Apply using VA Form 29-4364, Application for Service-Disabled Veterans Life Insurance.
You can download this form from the forms page on the insurance website at www.insurance.va.gov.

For more information about S-DVI, visit www.insurance.va.gov or call the VA Insurance Service toll-free at 800-669-8477.

Waiver of S-DVI Premiums (VA Form 29-357)

S-DVI policyholders who have a mental or physical disability that prevents them from performing substantially gainful employment may be eligible for waiver of premiums. The policyholder's disability must begin before their sixty-fifth birthday and must continue for at least six consecutive months.

To apply for waiver of premiums, you must file VA Form 29-357, Claim for Disability Insurance Benefits, available for download from the forms page at www.insurance.va.gov. For more information about waiver of S-DVI premiums, visit www.insurance.va.gov, or call the VA Insurance Service toll-free at 800-669-8477.

Supplemental S-DVI (VA Form 29-0188)

Supplemental S-DVI provides $20,000 of supplemental coverage to S-DVI policyholders who are approved for waiver of premiums. Premiums may not be waived on this supplemental coverage.

S-DVI policyholders are eligible for this supplemental coverage if

- They are eligible for a waiver of premiums.
- They apply for the coverage within one year from notice of the grant of waiver of premiums.
- They are under age sixty-five.

To apply for Supplemental S-DVI, you must

- File VA Form 29-0188, Application for Supplemental Service-Disabled Veterans (RH) Life Insurance, OR
- Send a signed letter requesting this insurance

You must apply for the coverage within one year from notice of the grant of waiver of premiums.

For more information about Supplemental S-DVI, visit www.insurance.va.gov or call the VA Insurance Service toll-free at 800-669-8477.

Veterans Mortgage Life Insurance (VA Form 29-8636)

The Veterans Mortgage Life Insurance (VMLI) program provides mortgage life insurance to severely disabled veterans. It is designed to pay off home mortgages of disabled veterans in the event of their death. If you have received a Specially Adapted Housing Grant from VA, you are eligible for VMLI. This is a grant to help you build or modify a home to accommodate your disabilities.

VMLI provides up to $90,000 of mortgage life insurance payable to the mortgage holder (i.e., a bank or mortgage lender) in the event of your death. This coverage reduces as the amount of your mortgage is reduced. A Specially Adapted Housing Agent will provide you with VA Form 29-8636, Veterans Mortgage Life Insurance Statement, and help you with the application process. You can also download the application at www.insurance.va.gov. For more information about VMLI, visit www.insurance.va.gov or call the VA Insurance Service toll-free at 800-669-8477.

Education Benefits

VA Education Benefits (VA Form 22-1990) allows you to apply for multiple education benefits, including the Montgomery G.I. Bill Educational Assistance Program, Montgomery G.I. Bill Selected Reserve Educational Assistance Program, Reserve Educational Assistance Program, Post-Vietnam Era Veterans Educational Assistance Program, National Call to Serve Program, and the Transfer of Entitlement Program.

Survivors' and Dependents' Educational Assistance (VA Form 22-5490)

This VA program provides for educational assistance to your spouse or child if you are permanently and totally disabled as a result of a service-connected disability, if you die due to a service-connected disability or while rated permanently and totally disabled, or if you are missing in action or a prisoner of war. The program offers up to forty-five months of education benefits. These benefits may be used for degree and certificate programs, apprenticeship, and on-the-job training. If you are a spouse, you may take a correspondence course. Remedial, deficiency, and refresher courses may be approved under certain circumstances. You can get more information on the program at https://www.gibill.va.gov.

Vocation and Education Counseling (VA Form 28-8832)

This program provides professional and qualified vocational and educational counseling to you and your family members who are eligible for educational benefits under a program that VA administers. You are eligible if you are discharged or released from active duty under honorable conditions not more than one year before date of application or if you are on active duty and have six or fewer months remaining before your scheduled release or discharge from service.

Vehicle Purchase and Adaptation (VA Form 21-4502)

This application can provide a one-time grant toward the purchase of a vehicle with adaptive equipment approved by VA for you, whether you are a veteran or service member, if you possess one of the following disabilities as a result of injury or disease incurred or aggravated during active military service: permanent loss of use of one or both hands or permanent loss of use of one or both feet, or permanent impairment of vision in both eyes. Entitlement to adaptive equipment may only be authorized with VA approval.

Housing Adaptation (VA Form 26-4555)

This application can provide grants for constructing an adapted home or modifying an existing home to meet your needs if you are a disabled veteran/ service member, in order to provide a barrier-free environment. For information on this program, visit the VA webpage at www.homeloans.va.gov/ sah.htm.

Clothing Allowance (VA Form 10-8678)

If you, because of a service-connected disability, wear or use prosthetics or an orthopedic appliance (including a wheelchair) that wears out or tears your clothing, or if you, because of a service-connected skin condition, use medication that causes irreparable damage to your garments, you can receive an annual clothing allowance.

For information regarding VA health benefits, go to chapter 7. Veteran benefits under the Department of Veterans Affairs are authorized under Title 38 of United States Code. You can get an in-depth explanation of VA benefits online at www.vba.va.gov/VBA/benefits/factsheets/index.asp or you can review the latest VA Benefits Handbook at www1.va.gov/OPA/publications/ benefits_book.asp to see all program information. All of the VA forms are available at www.va.gov/vaforms/.

SOCIAL SECURITY BENEFITS

Like many military members, you are probably aware that benefits are available from DoD and VA sources, but you may not be aware that the Social Security Administration (SSA) also may be able to provide you disability benefits if your medical conditions will cause a severe impact on your ability to work.

SSA benefits are different from those from the Department of Veterans Affairs and require a separate application. If you are an active military service member and became disabled on or after October 1, 2001, regardless of where your injuries occurred, you are eligible for expedited processing of disability benefits from the SSA.

What Types of Benefits Can Service Members Receive?

The SSA pays disability benefits through two programs:

- Social Security Disability Insurance Program (SSDI)
- Supplemental Security Income (SSI)

For you or your family to receive SSDI benefits, you have to be considered "insured" by the SSA. This means you have worked long enough and paid enough Social Security taxes to meet the eligibility for benefits. In order to receive SSI benefits a financial need must be demonstrated. For more information about Social Security's disability program, go to www.socialsecurity .gov/woundedwarriors.

What Is Social Security's Definition of Disability?

- You must be unable to do substantial work because of your medical condition(s).
- Your medical condition(s) must have lasted, or be expected to last, at least one year or be expected to result in death.

Social Security does not pay money for partial disabilities or short-term disabilities.

How Does Military Pay Affect Eligibility for Disability Benefits?

Being on active duty or getting military pay does not automatically prevent you from receiving Social Security benefits. You should still apply for Social Security if you think you are disabled. If you are receiving treatment from a military treatment facility (MTF) and are working in a designated therapy program or are on limited duty, Social Security will evaluate your work activity to determine your eligibility for benefits (the actual work activity is the controlling factor—not the amount of pay you receive or your military status).

How Do You Apply for Benefits?

You can apply for disability benefits while in the military or after separating from the military.

This also applies if you are still hospitalized, in a rehabilitation program, or undergoing outpatient treatment in an MTF or civilian medical facility. You may apply online at www.socialsecurity.gov/woundedwarriors (there is a starter kit that is available at this website to help you complete your application) or in person at the nearest Social Security Office. Or, you can call 800-772-1213 (TTY 800-325-0778) between the hours of 7 a.m. and 7 p.m. to schedule an appointment.

What Do I Need to Apply?

You or your representative must provide proof of identity to include

- Proof of age
- Proof of U.S. citizenship or legal residency, if foreign born
- Form DD214, if discharged from the military service
- W-2 Form or income tax return from the previous year
- Military or worker's compensation to include proof of payment
- Social Security numbers of your spouse and minor children
- Checking or savings account number, if you have one
- Name, address, and phone number of a contact person, in case you are unavailable
- Medical records that you may have and/or that you can easily obtain from all military and civilian sources

Important: File your application for disability benefits as soon as possible with available documentation. Do not delay your filing because you do not have all of your documentation.

How Does Social Security Make a Decision to Pay a Claim?

Your claim is handled by the state Disability Determination Services (DDS) office that makes disability decisions. Medical and vocational experts from the DDS will contact your physicians where you receive treatment, in order to retrieve your medical records. The DDS may ask you to have an examination or medical test. You will not have to pay for these exams or tests.

How Long Does It Take for a Decision?

The length of time to receive a decision on your disability claim could vary. It depends on

- The nature of your disability
- How quickly the DDS office obtains medical evidence from your doctor or medical sources
- Whether it is necessary to send you for a medical examination in order to obtain evidence to support your claim

What Can I Do to Expedite the Process?

You can expedite the process by being prepared for your interview. It also helps to have information regarding your work history and physicians who have treated you.

After your claim is received by the DDS, it is uniquely identified as a military service member claim, and it is expedited through all phases of processing both at the SSA and the DDS. Disability claims that have been filed online are also expedited.

Note: You can prevent delays by notifying SSA of any change in address or if you are being seen or treated by any new doctors, hospitals, or clinics while they are working on your claim.

Can My Family Receive Benefits?

Certain members of your family may qualify for benefits based on your employment history.

They include

- Your spouse, if he or she is sixty-two years or older.
- Your spouse at any age, if he or she is caring for a child of yours who is younger than sixteen or disabled.
- Your unmarried child, including an adopted child, or in some cases, a stepchild or grandchild. The child must be younger than eighteen years of age or younger than nineteen if in elementary school or secondary school.
- Your unmarried child, age eighteen or older, if he or she has a disability that started before age twenty-two (the child's disability must meet the definition of disability for adults).

Note: In some cases, a divorced spouse may qualify for benefits based on your earnings if he or she was married to you for at least ten years, is not currently married, and is at least sixty-two years of age. The money paid to a divorced spouse does not reduce your benefit or any benefit due to your current spouse or children.

How Can I Contact Social Security?

For more information and publications, visit www.socialsecurity.gov or call toll-free: 800-772-1213 (TTY: 800-325-0778) between the hours of 7 a.m. and 7 p.m. to schedule an appointment. All calls are treated confidentially and Social Security representatives are monitoring telephone calls to ensure that the information you receive is accurate and delivered in a courteous manner.

RESOURCES REGARDING BENEFITS

Pay and Allowances

Army Travel Pay Webpage at DFAS

Visit the Army's website at www.dfas.mil/travelpay/armytravelpay.html to learn about their travel pay services.

Marine Corps Casualty Branch

Contact the Marine Corps Casualty Branch at 800-847-1597 to learn about the marine travel pay services.

Air Force

Call the Air Force at 800-433-0048 to get more information on their policies for travel pay.

Navy

Contact your Safe Harbor representative to get details on how to get family travel allowances.

DFAS Travel Pay Questions/Answers

For general travel information for all branches, visit www.dfas.mil/travelpay.html or call 888-332-7366.

DFAS Disability Retirement Webpage

To learn about the different kinds of Disability Retirements, visit www.dfas.mil/militarypay/woundedwarriorpay/disabilityretirements.html.

DFAS Wounded Warrior Homepage

To learn about different aspects of Wounded Warrior pay services such as casual pay, pay allowance, travel, and the Savings Deposit Program, visit www.dfas.mil/militarypay/woundedwarriorpay.html.

Title 10, Chapter 71, Section 1401

You can go to http://uscode.house.gov/download/title_10.shtml to view the U.S. Code.

Traumatic Servicemembers' Group Life Insurance (TSGLI)

Army

For information on the Army's TSGLI program, visit https://www.hrc
.army.mil/site/crsc/tsgli/index.html, or e-mail TSGLI@conus.army.mil, or
call 800-237-1336 and press option 2 for TSGLI.

Army National Guard

To learn about the Army National Guard's TSGLI program, go to https://
www.hrc.army.mil/site/crsc/tsgli/index.html, or e-mail raymond.holdeman
@ng.army.mil, or call 703-607-5851.

Navy

Information about the Navy's TSGLI program is available at www.npc
.navy.mil/CommandSupport/CasualtyAssistance/TSGLI, or you can e-mail
MILL_TSGLI@navy.mil, or call 800-368-3202.

Marine Corps

The Marine Corps TSGLI website is located at https://www.manpower
.usmc.mil/portal/page?_pageid = 278,3206641&_dad = portal&_schema =
PORTAL, or for more information you can e-mail t-sgli@usmc.mil, or call
877-216-0825.

Air Force

To learn about the Air Force's TSGLI program, e-mail afpc.casualty@ran
dolph.af.mil, or call 210-565-3505.

Air Force Reserves

Information about the Air Force Reserves TSGLI program is available by
calling 800-525-0102, Ext. 227.

Air National Guard

To learn about the Air National Guard's TSGLI program, call 703-607-
1239.

Coast Guard

The Coast Guard's TSGLI information is available by calling 202-475-
5391, faxing 202-475-5927, or e-mailing comdt@compensation.uscg.mil or
terrence.w.walsh@uscg.mil.

Family and Medical Leave Act (FMLA)

How It Applies to You

To learn about how the FMLA can apply to you, visit www.dol.gov/whd/fmla/index.htm.

National Defense Authorization Act (NDAA) Changes to FMLA

For information on how the NDAA changes apply to the FMLA, you can go to www.dol.gov/whd/fmla/NDAA_fmla.htm.

Law Amended with NDAA Input

To view the FMLA with the amended NDAA input, go to www.dol.gov/whd/fmla/fmlaAmended.htm.

Public Law 10-181 (2008 NDAA)

To read the public law, go to frwebgate.access.gpo.gov/cgi-bin/getdoc .cgi?dbname = 110_cong_public_law s&docid = f:publ181.110.pdf.

Department of Labor

Department of Labor Wage and Hour Helpline

For information on federal regulations of minimum wage, overtime pay, and more, call 866-487-9243 or visit www.dol.gov/whd/index.htm.

State Listing of DOL Wage and Hour Division Office Contacts

To view state-specific contact information for DOL Wage and Hour Division (WHD) offices across the country go to www.dol.gov/dol/location.htm.

VA Benefits

Description of VA Benefits

For a basic description of VA benefits, visit www.vba.va.gov/VBA/benefits/factsheets/index.asp or call 800-827-1000.

VA Forms

For a searchable collection of VA forms, go to www.va.gov/vaforms or call 800-827-1000 for more information.

VA Online Applications

You can now apply for many VA benefits through an online application process. Visit www.va.gov/onlineapps.htm for more information.

Social Security Administration (SSA) Benefits

SSA Wounded Warriors Benefits

You can go to www.socialsecurity.gov/woundedwarriors or call 800-772-1213 to learn about the SSA benefits available to Wounded Warriors.

Nonmedical Support

By now, you've probably noticed that the bulk of your medical care is being handled by a group of professionals and that a person with the title PEBLO, or Physical Evaluation Board Liaison Officer, has contacted you to help you understand where you are in the DES process and what to expect.

But did you know that you and your family members have access to support in a variety of other forms? Are you aware that your service has a specific program that assigns an advocate to you for the entire time you are going through this process—and beyond?

Do you need a permanent wheelchair ramp built to your home's front door? There are organizations that can help you get that ramp built. Do you need help with your resume just in case you have to leave the service? What about free or partly subsidized quality child care for visits to the hospital? There are organizations in place that can help you with both.

There are countless government and nongovernment organizations and agencies that consider it an honor to do their part to assist you and your family during this difficult time. This section will introduce you to a number of them and give you websites, phone numbers, and e-mail addresses to contact them directly.

Vet Centers

The Department of Veterans Affairs, Veterans Health Administration Vet Center program operates a system of 232 community-based counseling centers staffed by small multidisciplinary teams of dedicated providers, many of whom are combat veterans themselves. Vet Centers provide individual, group, and family counseling to all veterans who served in any combat zone. This service is provided free of charge to you and your family members.

Vet Centers offer readjustment counseling—a wide range of services provided to combat veterans in the effort to help make the transition from military to civilian life go more smoothly. Services include individual and group counseling, marital and family counseling, bereavement counseling, medical referrals, assistance in applying for VA benefits, employment counseling, guidance and referral, alcohol and drug abuse assessments, information about and referral to community resources, counseling and referral for sexual trauma that happened while serving in the military, and outreach and community education.

A service member or veteran who served in any combat zone and received a military campaign ribbon (Vietnam, Southwest Asia, OEF, OIF, etc.), or their family members, is eligible for Vet Center services.

Call them toll-free during normal business hours at 800-905-4675 (Eastern) and 866-496-8838 (Pacific). You can locate a Vet Center near you by going to their website at www.vetcenter.va.gov.

Veterans Service Organizations

In addition to the assistance available through the VA, there are many VSOs that can provide assistance and advice to service members, veterans, and their families on applying for or accessing VA benefits. Chapter 11 includes a list of many of the VSOs that are chartered by Congress and/or recognized by VA for claims representation for today's returning service members, veterans, and their families. A complete listing of all chartered and nonchartered VSOs is available online at www1.va.gov/vso/index.cfm.

Recovery Coordinator

Your Recovery Coordinator's goal is to help make sure you get the right care and support from the right people at the right time. He or she is trained to help build a Recovery Plan, which lays out the path for you to meet personal and professional goals during your recovery. Your Recovery Coordinator will work with the doctors, nurses, social workers, and service-specific Wounded Warrior program staff to create the Recovery Plan and put it into action.

A key part of this Recovery Plan is identifying, applying for, and receiving the right benefits and compensation. Your Recovery Coordinator will provide oversight and assistance, identifying any gaps in your nonclinical services and intervening as necessary to expedite outcomes that will help you

find and connect with federal, state, local, nonprofit, and private-sector programs that offer you the support and benefits you and your family need.

Sometimes your Recovery Coordinator will be in the same location as you,
and sometimes your Recovery Coordinator will be available by phone or
e-mail. Either way, that person is someone you can trust as your ultimate
resource for information and assistance.

Legal and Financial Counseling

Specific counseling is often needed when the recovering service member
can't manage his or her own legal and financial affairs. If your loved one has
not been medically retired and is still considered "in the military," then the
nearest military installation probably has a legal service office that can assist
you both with powers of attorney, will preparation, and legal advice, to name
just a few of their services. Sometimes these services are also available to retirees on a case-by-case basis.

Another way to locate an attorney is through an attorney referral service.
The Bar Association in your community may have a panel that refers callers
to lawyers in various specializations. Initial consultations generally include
a nominal fee. Visit their site at www.abanet.org/legalservices/findlegalhelp/
home.cfm.

Transportation Services

The Americans with Disabilities Act requires transit agencies to provide
curb-to-curb paratransit service to those individuals who are unable to use
regular public transportation. Paratransit generally consists of wheelchair-ac-
cessible vans or taxis for people with disabilities and is run by private, nonprofit, and/or public organizations and is usually free or low-cost. To learn
more about paratransit near you, call Project Action, which maintains a national paratransit database, at 800-659-6428 or 202-347-3066. You can view
the database at.projectaction.easterseals.com/site/PageServer?pagename = ES
PA_rel_links.

Respite Care

Respite care is an option for those who need relief from the demands of
providing constant care for the recovering service member. It gives the regular caregiver some time off to breathe, relax, and regroup. Respite care reduces caregiver stress and can allow the caregiver to do activities that may

also relieve some sadness. Respite care includes adult day care and homecare services, as well as overnight stays in a facility, and can be provided a few hours a week or for a weekend.

Many caregiver support programs offer respite assistance as part of their services. Some service organizations offer volunteer respite workers who provide companionship or protective supervision only.

Respite care may be available for active duty service members for qualifying medical conditions as determined by TRICARE. Qualifying conditions may include extraordinary physical or psychological conditions of such severity that they result in the service member being homebound with a primary caregiver necessary to assist with the activities of daily living. To determine eligibility, contact your primary care provider or TRICARE directly.

Another option for assistance is to contact the appropriate military aid/relief services—Army Emergency Relief (AER), Navy Marine Corps Relief Society (NMCRS), and Air Force Aid Society (AFAS). These organizations can assist you with respite care, although you will need to contact them to make sure you understand any limits they may have. Some limits might include a financial cap and whether or not the recovering service member is still active duty. You may also obtain information about these programs through your installation Family Support Center or Airman and Family Readiness Center. Additionally, the NMCRS offers the Visiting Nurse service.

Respite care may be provided by:

- Home health care workers
- Adult day care centers
- Short-term nursing homes
- Assisted living homes

For more information regarding being a caregiver or getting support, including respite care, call the National Women's Health Information Center at 800-994-9662 or contact the following organizations:

National Respite Locator Service: Call them at 800-773-5433. Or visit their website at archrespite.org/respitelocator.

Administration for Children and Families: Call them at 202-401-9215. Or visit their website at www.acf.hhs.gov.

National Adult Day Services Association: Call them at 877-745-1440. Or visit their website at www.nadsa.org.

National Family Caregivers Association: Call them at 800-896-3650. Or
visit their website at www.nfcacares.org.

National Family Caregivers Support Program (Administration on Aging):
Call them at 202-619-0724. Or visit their website at www.aoa.gov/.

Adult Day Care and Adult Social Day are programs more often available for
the elderly, but the organizations that offer these services may also be able to
assist you. The National Adult Day Services Association can help you find
adult day care services that are suitable for your loved one's needs. Visit their
site at www.nadsa.org or call them at 877-745-1440.

Home Care is generally categorized as home health care services and com-
bines health care and supportive services to help homebound sick or disabled
persons continue living at home as independently as possible. There are two
types of home care available to you: home health care services and nonmedical home care services. Home health care services provide a range of medical
services, including medication assistance, nursing services, and physical therapy. You may not need this assistance while your recovering service member
is still affiliated with the MTF. However, depending upon the situation, home
health care may become very helpful. Nonmedical home care services include
companionship, housekeeping, cooking, and many other household activities
and chores.

The cost of these services depends on the level of care needed—a nonmedical home care attendant may charge less money than a nurse who is monitoring the person's condition and treatment. Fees vary so you may want to
shop around. Some private insurance policies pay for limited home health
care with certain restrictions. Check your TRICARE coverage to see what is
offered. In some cases, you may have to pay out of pocket. When that's the
case, remember to turn to the NMCRS, Army Emergency Relief (AER), or
AFAS to request financial assistance. They may be able to provide temporary
help. See Financial Assistance (below) for more information regarding these
organizations.

Nonmedical home care aides can be located through personal referrals or
at a private home care agency, hospital, social service agency, public health
department or other community organizations.

In some areas, nursing schools may be of assistance.

The National Association for Home Care and Hospice (www.nahc.org)
can assist with finding the right provider. The site includes a comprehensive

database of more than 20,000 home care and hospice agencies and walks you through the process to find the right care resource for your needs.

Financial Assistance

NMCRS, AFAS, and AER can offer financial assistance in a number of cases. For more information regarding what is available to help you and your loved one, contact the appropriate organization below:

Air Force Aid Society: www.afas.org/ or call them at 800-769-8951.
Navy-Marine Corps Relief Society: www.nmcrs.org/ or call them at 703-696-4904. For a more local number, select the location nearest you from the map located on this webpage: www.nmcrs.org/locations.html.
Army Emergency Relief: www.aerhq.org/index.asp or call them at 866-878-6378.

Support Groups

Support Groups are a good source of information on available resources. Support groups provide caregivers with the opportunity to give and receive encouragement, understanding, and support from others who have similar concerns. Interacting with other caregivers can be a great help in reducing stress. Support groups can be found through hospitals, mental health programs, and military aid and injured support programs. There are also online support groups available to caregivers with computer access. Family Caregiver Alliance offers a caregiver support group at www.caregiver.org/caregiver/jsp/content_node.jsp?nodeid = 486.

Employee Assistance Programs are an employment benefit that your workplace may or may not offer. Assistance varies widely, though programs generally provide employees with counseling for personal issues such as depression, stress, addiction, financial crisis, and illness or death in the family. If you are enrolled in TRICARE Prime, you may be covered for a number of mental health visits. Visit their site and take the self-assessment to determine if you could benefit from treatment or evaluation: www.tricare.mil/my benefit/home/MentalHealthAndBehavior/GettingHelp.

Assistance with Your Resource Search

It's a confusing and painful time for you. Contacting the resources for assistance can be a time-consuming job, but it's worthwhile. Your PEBLO, service-provided advocate, or Recovery Coordinator will be able to help you locate resources, as well.

The following is a list of suggestions to help you find appropriate services:

- Begin looking for resources right away, even if you don't think you'll need them. This way, you'll be better informed to make important decisions during a time of crisis.
- Understand that there may be a waiting list for some of the services you'd like. This is one of the reasons it's best to ask for help before you think you'll actually need it.
- Write down all of the information you are given or find. Document the name of each agency you called, the phone number or website, the names of the people you spoke with, the date of your conversations, the services requested, the services promised, and any agreed-upon decisions.
- Don't hang up until you understand the next step, for instance, who calls whom next, what will be done next, and so on.
- When you make your call, be prepared with specific information, such as physician's name, diagnostic information, insurance coverage, and Social Security numbers.
- When dealing with agencies, be specific about your needs.
- Don't hesitate to ask for help. Most community agencies are there specifically to provide support to those who need it. Many of the services you've paid for with your taxes, service fees, and contributions.
- Not everyone you call will understand what you are going through or what your needs are. You may need to spend some time educating the person on the other end of the phone. Doing this will help you get the services you need.
- Be persistent!

SUPPORT PROGRAMS

There are many military, government, and nongovernment agencies available to assist you and your family in your recovery, rehabilitation, and reintegration. In this section, you'll find many of them, along with a short description of the support available, as well as phone numbers, when available, and web addresses.

Government Support

Military Severely Injured Center

Navigating through the military and government programs to find assistance for service members who are severely injured can be a real challenge. One way to overcome the hurdles is to contact the DoD Military Severely Injured Center (MSIC) and let them help.

When you call them at 888-774-1361, you will talk to an actual human being who will provide assistance with a variety of services, including medical care and rehabilitation; education, training, and job placement; personal mobility and functioning; home, transportation, and workplace accommodations; individual, couple, and family counseling; and financial resources.

The counselor advocates assigned to MSIC have master's degrees in counseling. Plus, each has received extensive training during a five-week MSIC session.

Besides the support received through the MSIC, an ombudsman is assigned to or near a major military facility or VA medical facility to further assist in the transition by helping you connect with local agencies and community groups.

Each service has its own program to assist severely injured service members and their families. The Army has the United States Army Wounded Warrior Program (AW2). The Marines offer the Wounded Warrior Regiment/ Marine for Life Injured Support Program. The Navy has the Navy Safe Harbor Program and the Air Force runs the Air Force Wounded Warrior Program (AFW2).

Army Wounded Warrior Program (AW2)

The AW2 Program's mission is to provide personalized support for the severely injured no matter where they are located or how long their recovery takes. AW2 advocates are located at MTFs and at VA medical facilities. They are considered career and education guides, benefits advisors, transition counselors, resource experts, family assistants, and life coaches. There are specific conditions that the soldier must meet to be qualified to receive the assistance of the AW2 Program. To learn more about those conditions, go to their website at aw2portal.com/ and click on their FAQs link near the top of the page.

The site offers opinions and stories from various people in its blog section.

There is also a link for opportunities specifically for members of the AW2 Program, as well as a link to My Benefits.

Wounded Warrior Regiment/Marine for Life Injured Support Program

The mission of the Wounded Warrior Regiment/Marine for Life Injured Support Program is to "provide information, advocacy and assistance to injured Marines, Sailors injured while serving with Marines, and their families, in order to minimize the difficulties and worries they face as they navigate the stressful and confusing process." Support begins at the time of the injury and continues until the service member returns to active duty or transitions to the VA.

The site includes a user-friendly Injured Support Process graph that allows you to click on each stage—from injury to follow-on treatment and rehabilitation to post-separation care. Each stage offers helpful, easy-to-understand information that very often also includes a phone number and a name of a person you can talk to if you have questions. Of particular interest is the information regarding family travel. Immediate family (up to three people) can get roundtrip tickets, arranged by the Casualty Assistance Section, to the bedside of the injured service member. (This information is also covered in depth earlier in this chapter.)

To learn more, go to the Marine for Life website at https://www.m4l.usmc.mil and click on the purple icon that reads, "Injured Marines and Sailors."

Navy Safe Harbor—Severely Injured Support

The Navy's program for the severely injured is run through the Navy Personnel Command and provides personalized assistance to severely injured sailors and their families. An advocate will contact the severely injured sailor once he or she reaches a stateside hospital and will assist in obtaining the resources needed to meet the identified nonmedical needs.

The site includes a "Roadmap to Recovery" that walks you through each step of the process—from the injury to convalescent leave, veteran status, and post-separation care. Each stage offers helpful, easy-to-understand information that very often also includes a phone number and a name of a person you can talk to if you have questions. Like the Marine site, there is information regarding family travel. Immediate family (up to three people) can get roundtrip tickets, arranged by the Casualty Assistance Section, to the bedside of the injured service member.

To learn more about the Navy's Safe Harbor program, go to their website at www.npc.navy.mil/safeharbor.

Air Force Wounded Warrior (AFW2) Program

The AFW2 Program (formerly known as Air Force Palace HART) provides a multifaceted support system that includes the assignment of a Family Liaison Officer and a Community Readiness Consultant through all phases of the recovery process, as needed. They will also assist in retention of disabled airmen from OEF and OIF whenever possible. Expanded transition assistance, extended case management follow-up, advocacy, and tracking are also part of the program. The AFW2 program is located at Headquarters Air Force Personnel Center on Randolph Air Force Base in San Antonio, Texas, and works hand-in-hand with Air Force installation Airman & Family Readiness Centers (A&FRCs) to ensure face-to-face, personalized services to wounded warriors. A&FRCs provide hands-on professional services such as transition assistance, employment assistance, moving assistance, financial counseling, information and referral, and emergency financial assistance, to name a few.

The AFW2 program advocates for services on an airman's behalf and ensures airmen have professional support and follow-up for no less than five years after separation or retirement. For more information about the AFW2 Program, call their toll-free number 800-581-9437 between 7 a.m. and 4 p.m. (Central time), send an e-mail to afwounded.warrior@randolph.af.mil, or visit the AFW2 website at www.woundedwarrior.af.mil.

Air Force Survivor Assistance Program

The Survivor Assistance Program provides immediate assistance to wounded airmen and their family members by the assignment of Family Liaison Officers. Call 877-USAF-HELP (877-872-3435) any time for support and/or referral to agencies that serve wounded airmen.

Army Knowledge Online (AKO)

Army Knowledge Online (AKO) is the U.S. Army's main intranet. It serves registered users to include active duty and retired service personnel and their family members, and provides single-sign-on access to over three hundred applications and services. It allows access to all of the personnel functions, so it's the place to go when you need a copy of something from your record. It allows you to fill out your assignment request forms to move to a new duty station or volunteer for a special assignment (airborne, Ranger, etc.). It is where you go to access your Army e-mail account. It includes your medical alerts—for instance when you are due for shots/physicals. It has the only authorized "chat" client for Army computers and it also has a video chat so troops who are deployed can log on and chat with their families. The website is www.us.army.mil.

Military Homefront

Military Homefront is the official DoD website for reliable quality-of-life information designed to help troops and their families, leaders, and service providers. There are useful links to programs such as Heroes to Hometowns—a program that is run at the state level and is the link among the services and VA case workers at the military and VA hospitals, severely injured service members, their families, and their local communities. Support has included help paying bills, finding suitable homes and adapting them as needed, adapting vehicles, finding transportation to medical appointments, finding jobs and providing educational assistance, locating child care support, and much more. Also on this site, you can find a glossary link that will give you access to not only their own glossary, but glossaries for the DoD and TRICARE. There are also links to fact sheets for every service. The website can be found at www.militaryhomefront.dod.mil/.

MyArmyBenefits

This site produces personalized survivor and retirement benefit reports for active duty service personnel and their family members. It provides a complete financial forecast that includes your investments, insurance, and SGLI. It also provides a "what if" capability that shows how life events, such as getting married, having children, or retiring at a projected date and rank, affect your financial picture.

If you aren't a soldier, you can still gain access to recent benefit news and updates, access a state-by-state listing of benefit resources, and benefit facts by category, component, and life event. It also provides fact sheets on various programs/agencies. The website can be found at myarmybenefits.us.army.mil.

TRICARE

TRICARE Online is the entry point that offers beneficiaries access to available health care services, benefits, and information. It has convenient tabs for medical care, dental care, vision care, prescriptions, mental health, and more. You can set up your own profile, learn about the different TRICARE programs, and compare the plans. You can also use the site to find a provider. The website can be found at www.tricare.mil. You can go to www.tricare.mil/contactus for a list of phone numbers for specific issues and locations.

Disability.gov

Disability.gov is the federal government's one-stop website for people with disabilities, their families, employers, veterans and service members, workforce professionals, and many others.

The site provides quick and easy access to comprehensive information about disability programs, services, laws, and benefits in areas including education, employment, housing, transportation, health, benefits, technology, community health, and civil rights.

The website can be found at www.disability.gov. For specific questions related to federal disability programs, you can call 800-FED-INFO (800-333-4636, voice and TTY) Monday–Friday, 8 a.m. to 8 p.m. Eastern time.

GovBenefits.gov

GovBenefits.gov is the official benefits website of the U.S. government, with information on over one thousand benefit and assistance programs. It provides information, fact sheets, and other resources for military personnel, family members, and veterans. You can fill in a questionnaire and the site will generate a list of benefit programs that could assist you. You can also target a specific benefit and learn more about it. The website can be found at www.govbenefits.gov/. You can also reach them at 800-FED-INFO (800-333-4636) Monday–Friday, 8 a.m. to 8 p.m. Eastern time.

America Supports You (ASY)

Their website is now incorporated into www.ourmilitary.mil, which provides links to hundreds of organizations eager to help service members and their families. If you click on "Want to request military support?" you will be directed to pages that list ways to receive help. Military OneSource

Military OneSource is a user-friendly site for military members and their families that can connect them to information regarding everything from being a caregiver to someone with disabilities, finding a job, to coping with post-traumatic stress. The site includes discussion boards on nearly every topic of concern to military and family members and access to in-person and phone counseling with master's-level consultants trained to provide confidential support and practical solutions. In addition, a Wounded Warrior Resource Center is being established to provide further information and assistance.

If you are qualified to become a member (active duty, Guard, Reserve, family members, and more) you can have access to more information, including financial calculators, interactive tools, locators for child care, summer camp, and the like, webinar access and free handbooks and informative CDs. During tax season, you can access free income tax software to assist in preparing your taxes. Phones are answered 24 hours a day, 7 days a week, and staff can make sure you get the information you need. Call them at 800-342-9647 and visit the site at www.militaryonesource.com.

Nongovernment Support

The sites included below are in no way meant as a complete list of nongovernmental support sites available, and their inclusion does not imply endorsement. However, you may find the following sites useful.

Heroes to Hometown—American Legion

The American Legion, working closely with MSIC, has created a program that actively engages the community in helping the returning severely injured service member. The program identifies and coordinates community resources with the desired outcome of a seamless support system. Assistance can include child care, transportation, shopping, odd jobs around the house, securing temporary housing, if needed, job opportunities, and a safe haven at the local American Legion.

The program may already be in place within your community as there have been a number of severely injured service members who have returned to their hometowns. If the program is not in place or if they have not contacted you, e-mail them at legion.h2h@itc.dod.mil, or call them at 703-692-2054.

National Association of Child Care Resource and Referral Agencies (NACCRRA)

If your spouse is a severely injured military member, you can get assistance from NACCRRA to find and pay for safe, licensed child care services for a period of six months during the service member's recuperation. You can get extensions beyond the six-month period based upon a physician reassessment. NACCRRA will coordinate with state and local agencies to help military families locate child care in the civilian community when a military program is unavailable. This will allow you to be at your spouse's bedside or there during medical appointments. NACCRRA and DoD will provide an offset to the civilian child care fees during the recovery period. The program is available nationwide wherever the injured service member is receiving either inpatient or outpatient medical care.

Go to www.naccrra.org/MilitaryPrograms/severely_injured/ to learn more and to begin the application process. Call Child Care Aware at 800-424-2246 for more information.

Rebuilding Together: National Initiatives—Veterans Housing

Rebuilding Together is a national nonprofit organization with a network of nearly 225 affiliates across the United States. Their mission is to bring volunteers and communities together to rehabilitate the homes of low-income homeowners. They may be able to help with home repairs and modifications.

For more information, go to www.rebuildingtogether.org/section/initia tives/veteran_housing/apply, e-mail them at mtesauro@rebuildingtogether .org, or call them at 800-473-4229.

Transition

The Department of Veterans Affairs (VA) has maintained an active Transition Assistance Program and Disabled Transition Assistance Program (TAP/ DTAP) throughout the United States and around the world. Since the implementation of TAP/DTAP through the original legislation (P.L. 101-237) and the legislation that expanded TAP/DTAP (P.L. 101-510) VA has provided benefit information to separating service members and their families. VA encourages all separating service members to contact their respective Transition Centers to determine when the VA Transition Assistance Briefings are scheduled. These briefings provide information that will help you make the transition to civilian life easier by identifying many of the VA benefits available to you. You may find the locations of the briefing sites through the Department of Defense transition portal website. When the site comes up, click on the At Your Service link. Click on the Military Services Transition Assistance Locations link to locate the center nearest you. (www.dodtransportal.org/dav/lsn media/LSN/dodtransportal/)

Links to Other Information

National Center for PTSD

The mission of the National Center for PTSD (post-traumatic stress disorder) is to advance the clinical care and social welfare of America's veterans through research, education, and training in the science, diagnosis, and treatment of PTSD and stress-related disorders. (www.ptsd.va.gov/).

PTSD Specific to OEF/OIF Veterans

Information for clinicians, veterans, and family members. (www.ptsd.va .gov/index.asp)

Army Review Boards Agency

This agency offers discharge review and correction to military records such as the DD 214. Visit them at https://secureweb.hqda.pentagon.mil/ ACTS_Online/gui/Login.aspx?ReturnUrl = %2fACTS_Online%2fgui%2flan ding.aspx.

Grief and Bereavement

TRAUMATIC GRIEF: SYMPTOMATOLOGY AND TREATMENT IN THE WAR VETERAN

Ilona Pivar, Ph.D.

Symptoms of Grief Are Distinct from PTSD and Depression

Although research into the prevalence and intensity of grief symptoms in war veterans is limited, clinicians recognize the importance for veterans of grieving the loss of comrades. Grief symptoms can include sadness; longing; missing the deceased; nonacceptance of the death; feeling the death was unfair; anger; feeling stunned, dazed, or shocked; emptiness; preoccupation with thoughts and images of the deceased; loss of enjoyment; difficulties in trusting others; social impairments; and guilt concerning the circumstances of the death. Recent research results, although limited to one sample of Vietnam combat veterans in a residential rehabilitation unit for PTSD, have supported findings in the general bereavement literature that unresolved grief can be detected as a distress syndrome distinct from depression and anxiety. In this sample of combat veterans, grief symptoms were detected at very high levels of intensity thirty years post-loss. The intensity of symptoms experienced after thirty years was similar to that reported in community samples of grieving spouses and parents at six months post-loss. This supports clinical observations that unresolved grief, if left untreated, can continue unabated and increases the distress load of veterans. The existence of a distinct and intense set of grief symptoms indicates the need for clinical attention to grief in the treatment plan.

Attachment and Bonding Are Essential to Unit Cohesiveness

Bonds with unit members are described by many veterans as some of the closest relationships they have formed in their lives. During Vietnam, soldiers were rotated in and out of units on individual schedules. Nevertheless, the percentage of returning veterans with PTSD who also report bereavement-related distress is high. In the Iraq conflict, young service personnel and reservists have remained with their units throughout training and deployment. Levels of mutual trust and respect, unit cohesiveness, and affective bonding will have been further strengthened by the experiences of deployment. While bonding and attachment to the unit may result in some protection against subsequent development of PTSD, unresolved bereavement may be expected to be associated with increased distress over the lifespan unless these losses are acknowledged and grief symptoms treated on a timely basis.

Traumatic Grief

Traumatic grief refers to the experience of the *sudden loss* of a significant and close attachment. Having a close buddy, identification with service personnel in the unit, and experiencing multiple losses were the strongest predictors of grief symptoms in the above sample of Vietnam veterans. Other factors that may influence the development of prolonged grief syndrome include survivor guilt, feelings of powerlessness in not being able to prevent the death, anger at others who are thought to have caused the death, anger at oneself for committing a self-perceived error resulting in the death, tasks of survival in combat taking precedence over grieving, not being able to show emotional vulnerability, numbing and defending against overwhelming emotions, not having an opportunity in the field to acknowledge the death, and increased sense of vulnerability by seeing someone close killed. Factors important in the Iraq War may include exposure to significant numbers of civilian casualties, exposure to death from friendly fire or accidents resulting from massive and rapid troop movements, and concern about culpability for having caused death or harm to civilians in cities. These factors may contribute to experiences of shock, disbelief, and self-blame that increase risk of traumatic and complicated grief reactions.

Experiences That Can Influence the Development of Intense Grief: What We Learned from Vietnam

The sudden loss of attachments takes many forms in the war zone. Service personnel may experience overwhelming self-blame for events that are not under their control, including deaths during the chaos of firefights, accidents and failures of equipment, medical triage, and casualties from friendly fire.

The everyday infantryman from Vietnam lived his mistakes over and over again, perhaps in order to find some way of relieving pain and guilt from the death of friends. Many medics during Vietnam suffered tremendously when they were not able to save members of their unit, especially when they identified strongly with the men under their care. Pilots called in to fire close to troops were overcome with guilt when their ordnance hit American service personnel even while saving a majority of men. Officers felt unique responsibility for the subordinates under their care and suffered undue guilt and grief when results of combat were damaging. Those who worked closely with civilians were often shocked when they witnessed deaths of people with whom they had come to develop mutual trust. Deaths of civilian women and children were difficult to bear.

Many of these same experiences can be expected to affect combat troops in Iraq.

Normal vs. Pathological Grief

Bereavement is a universal experience. Intense emotions, including sadness, longing, anger, and guilt, are reactions to the loss of a close person. Common in the first days and weeks of grieving are intense emotions, usually experienced as coming in waves lasting twenty minutes to an hour, with accompanying somatic sensations in the stomach, tightness in the throat, shortness of breath, intense fatigue, feeling faint, agitation, and helplessness. Lack of motivation, loss of interest in outside activities, and social withdrawal are also fairly common. A person experiencing normal grief will have a gradual decline in symptoms and distress. When grief symptoms remain at severely discomforting levels, even after two months, a referral to a clinician can be considered. If intense symptoms persist after six months, a diagnosis of complicated grief can be made and there is a definite indication for clinical intervention. Complicated grief prolonged over time has been shown to have negative effects on health, social functioning, and mental health.

Acute Traumatic Grief

Survivors of traumatic events can experience acute symptoms of distress including intense agitation, self-accusations, high-risk behaviors, suicidal ideation, and intense outbursts of anger, superimposed on the symptoms of normal bereavement. Service personnel who lose their comrades in battle have been known to make heroic efforts to save them or recover their bodies.

Some have reacted with rage at the enemy, risking their lives with little thought ("gone berserk" or "kill crazy"). Some withdraw and become loners, seldom or never again making friends; some express extreme anger at the events and personnel that brought them to the conflict. Some are inclined to mask their emotions. Any sign of vulnerability or "losing it" can indicate that they are not tough enough to handle combat. Delaying grief may well postpone problems that can become chronic symptoms weeks, months, and years later. The returning veteran who has developed PTSD and/or depression may well be masking his or her grief symptoms.

Assessment and Treatment of Acute Grief in Returning Veterans

Clinical judgment is necessary in deciding when and how to treat acute grief reactions, especially when they are accompanied by a diagnosis of acute stress disorder. While a cognitive-behavioral treatment package that includes exposure therapy has been shown to prevent the development of PTSD in some persons with acute stress disorder, exposure therapy during the initial stages of grief may often be contraindicated, because it may place great emotional strain on someone only just bereaved. Bereavement researchers also are hesitant to treat grief in the first few months of a normal loss, wishing not to interfere with a natural healing process. In the early stages of grief, symptoms may be experienced as intense, but this is normal for the first days, weeks, and months. Those surviving a traumatic loss in the war zone will be more likely to mask intense feelings of sadness, pain, vulnerability, anxiety, anger, and guilt. Balancing other traumatic experiences with the intensity of grief may feel overwhelming. Therefore it is important to assess and respect the individual soldier's ability to cope and manage these feelings at any time. A soldier may be relieved to know that someone understands how he or she feels after losing a buddy, or experiencing other losses including civilians or multiple deaths in the field, and communication with a clinician may be a first step in coming to terms with loss. However, that soldier may not be ready to probe more deeply into feelings and circumstances. Care and patience in the assessment process, as well as in beginning treatment, is essential.

Treatment during the acute stages of grief would best include acknowledgment of the loss, communication of understanding of the depth of feelings, encouragement to recover positive memories of the deceased, recognition of the good intentions of the survivor to come to the aid of the deceased, education about what to expect during the course of acute grief, and encouragement of distraction and relaxation techniques as a temporary palliative. Efforts to reduce symptoms of PTSD and depression as comorbid disorders would take precedence over grief symptoms in the initial phases of treatment, unless the loss itself is the main cause of distress.

Assessment of Complicated Grief in Returning Veterans

Grief symptoms including sadness, distress, guilt, anger, intrusive thoughts, and preoccupation with the death should be declining after about six months during a normal grieving process. If symptoms remain very high after six months, clinical intervention is warranted. There are several instruments that may be helpful in assessing a complicated grief. The Inventory of Complicated Grief—Revised is perhaps most widely used and reflects current bereavement research. Another instrument is the Texas Revised Inventory of Grief, which has been used in a variety of populations and has been well validated. Both allow comparisons with normative populations.

Treatment of Complicated Grief in Returning Veterans

There have been no outcome studies of treatments of veterans for prolonged and complicated grief symptoms at this time. Clinical experience supports the importance of education about normal and complicated grief processes, education about the cognitive processes of guilt, restructuring of cognitive distortions of events that might lead to excessive guilt, looking at the function of anger in bereavement, restoring positive memories of the deceased, restoration and acknowledgment of caring feelings toward the deceased, affirming resilience and positive coping, retelling the story of the death, and learning to tolerate painful feelings as part of the grieving process. These activities can be provided in individual treatment or in closed groups.

Regardless of the techniques that are used, what is central to treating veterans for prolonged and complicated grief is recognition of the significance of their losses, provision of an opportunity to talk about the deceased, restructuring of distorted thoughts of guilt, and validation of the pain and intensity of their feelings. What is most essential is that bereavement and loss be treated in addition to PTSD and depression for a more complete recovery.

Medications Helpful in Treating Grief Symptoms in Nonveteran Populations

One research study has shown that paroxetine as well as nortriptyline may be helpful in treating complicated grief after six months. Bupropion has been successful in treating symptoms at six to eight weeks. Again, research has been limited and has not included war zone veterans.

HELPING BEREAVED MILITARY CHILDREN

Robin F. Goodman, Ph.D., Judith A. Cohen, M.D., and Stephen J. Cozza, M.D.

The joy of family reunion after a military deployment is often more than children or parents even hoped for. However, for some children the reunion never comes. Sadly, some children must cope with the death of a parent. There are often no words to console a child or explain what happened. But surviving family members, adults, and a caring community can help grieving military children. Below are some suggestions to help ease children's pain and support their resilience after a death.

- **Be honest and open**
  All children need information appropriate to their age. Use clear language that includes the term "death" rather than euphemisms (e.g., "loss," "gone to sleep") that may confuse children. Follow the child's lead and need for explanations of what happened. Rather than having just one conversation, stay open to ongoing questions and discussions.
- **Provide a sense of safety and security**
  Reestablishing routines and structure go a long way toward providing children a comforting sense of stability in the midst of changes. This can be done in the simplest of ways, for example, keeping up with ongoing after-school activities and regular bedtimes.
- **Be a good detective**
  Pay attention to how and what your child is communicating. Children often show their feelings and thoughts by their behaviors. Take a step back, ask the right questions, listen, and validate their feelings.
- **Support expression of feelings**
  Drawing, writing, playing, or reading books about grief can help children learn about and express feelings. Let them know all feelings are acceptable and help children find healthy ways to channel them.

- **Be a good role model**

  Children look to caregivers for examples of how to react and cope. It's okay for grownups to show their emotions, as long as they are not out of control or frightening to children. Adult expressions of sadness can model healthy ways of dealing with difficult feelings. For example, you can say: "I'm crying because I feel sad your dad is missing your soccer game; it's okay for you to cry when you miss him too."

- **Help children learn about the person and stay connected**

  Sharing stories, photos, and memories helps keep the person alive in the child's heart and keeps the person a part of the child's identity. For example, you can say: "Even though dad died, we can still remember how much fun we had together on our beach vacations."

- **Keep perspective about non-grief-related areas**

  Remember that children are still moving forward in their lives. Be aware of other developmental milestones and issues your children are facing at different ages, such as peer pressure or worry over school work, which may or may not relate to the person who died. Grief may make some of these times more difficult, for example, a teen not having his dad to teach him to drive.

- **Partner with other trusted adults in your child's world**

  Educate others about your child's grief and collaborate with them to support your child. For example, give and get feedback from teachers and coaches.

- **Look for peer support**

  Children and caregivers can benefit from being with others who "know what it's like." Some can benefit from groups that mix military and non-military families, others prefer military-specific groups such as those found on a base or offered by Tragedy Assistance Program for Survivors (TAPS), which holds Survivor Seminars and Good Grief Camps regionally across the country.

- **Take care of yourself**

  The better and stronger you are, the better caregiver you will be to your children. This includes taking care of your physical health (e.g., eating, sleeping, exercising, relaxing, etc.). This can also decrease children's worry about the people they depend on. Take care of your emotional health as well by managing stress and connecting to supportive friends and family who can help you.

- **Be alert to children who may be having difficulty**
  Some children may have a traumatic reaction. Some signs that children need more help include their being bothered by upsetting and recurring thoughts or images of the deceased person or the death, avoidance of military-related reminders or talk about the person who died, and unusual irritability or jumpiness. If you notice these behaviors in your child consider seeking professional help.
- **Seek professional support**
  Caregivers and children may believe they should be able to handle their grief on their own or that they are weak if they need help, and neither is true. Important communities to reach out for assistance include
  - school
  - community
  - medical
  - mental health
  - faith-based resources when needed

Grief is a new experience for many people. With any new experience, you can help to learn more about it, get answers to questions, and develop strategies to help you and your child get through it.

Resources

WEBSITES

- Real Warriors Campaign
- U.S. Department of Defense
- After Deployment
- Defense and Veterans Brain Injury Center
- Deployment Health Clinical Center
- TRICARE
- National Center for Post-traumatic Stress Disorder
- Center for the Study of Traumatic Stress
- Military Health System
- Force Health Protection and Readiness
- Military OneSource
- U.S. Department of Veterans Affairs
- Veterans Affairs' Mental Health Home
- Veterans Suicide Prevention Hotline
- National Resource Directory
- Army
- Army Behavioral Health
- Army OneSource
- Battlemind
- Hooah 4 Health's Deployment Information
- Army Wounded Warrior Program
- Ourmilitary.mil
- Comprehensive Soldier Fitness
- Navy
- Naval Center Combat & Operational Stress Control (NCCOSC)

- Navy and Marine Corps Public Health Center's "Minding Your Mental Health"
- Lifelines Services Network
- Navy Safe Harbor
- Marines Suicide Prevention
  Marine Corps Community Services Deployment Support
- Wounded Warrior Regiment
- Leaders Guide for Managing Marines in Distress
- Combat Stress Operational Control
- Air Force
- Air Force Crossroads
- Air Force Wounded Warriors
- Coast Guard
- OASD Reserve Affairs
- DoD Yellow Ribbon Reintegration Program
- Warfighter Brain Health Portal—Soldiers
- Warfighter Brain Health Portal—Providers
- NCIRE—The Veterans Health Research Institute
- Brainline.org
- American Veterans with Brain Injuries
- Warrior Gateway

REPORTS

- *Department of Veterans Affairs Office of Inspector General Follow-Up Healthcare Inspection*
- *The Health Care System for Veterans: An Interim Report*
- *TBI Task Force Report to the Surgeon General*
- *The Department of Defense Plan to Achieve the Vision of the DoD Task Force on Mental Health—Report to Congress*
- *An Achievable Vision: Report of the DoD Task Force on Mental Health*
- *Task Force on the Future of Military Health Care*
- *Report of the President's Commission on Care for America's Returning Wounded Warriors*
- *OIG Report on DoD/VA Care Transition Process for Service Members Injured in OIF/OEF*
- *Audit of Veterans Benefits Administration Transition Assistance for Operations Enduring and Iraqi Freedom Service Members and Veterans*

FACT SHEETS

- *Health Behaviors to Decrease Risk of Flu Transmission*
- *Mental Health and Behavioral Guidelines for Response to a Pandemic Flu Outbreak*
- *Mobilization and Demobilization Information and Resources Guide*
- *DVBIC Fact Sheet on Traumatic Brain Injury*

RESOURCES FOR FAMILIES

TBI Information

- CDC's National Center for Injury Prevention and Control: www.cdc.gov/ncipc/tbi/TBI.htm
- National Institute of Neurological Disorders and Stroke (NINDS) Traumatic Brain Injury Information Page: www.ninds.nih.gov/disorders/tbi/tbi.htm
- Traumatic Brain Injury National Resource Center: www.nrc.pmr.vcu.edu
- Brainline (DVBIC-sponsored): www.brainline.org
- Brain Injury Association of America: www.biausa.org

Wounded, Ill, and Injured

- Army Wounded Warrior (AW2) Program: aw2portal.com/Default.aspx
- USMC Wounded Warrior Regiment: https://www.manpower.usmc.mil/portal/page?_pageid = 278,3065271 &_dad = por tal&_schema = PORTAL
- Navy Safe Harbor: www.npc.navy.mil/CommandSupport/SafeHarbor/
- Air Force Wounded Warrior (AFW2): www.woundedwarrior.af.mil/

Transition Assistance

- TurboTap: www.transitionassistanceprogram.com/register.tpp
- DoD TransPortal: www.dodtransportal.dod.mil
- MyHealtheVet: www.myhealth.va.gov/mhv-portal-web
- Social Security Benefits for Wounded Warriors: www.ssa.gov/woundedwarriors

Caregivers

- Family Caregiver Alliance—National Center on Caregiving: www.caregiving.org/
- National Alliance for Caregiving: www.caregiver.org

- Health and Human Services—Medicare Site—Caregiving Exchange: www
  .medicare.gov/caregivers/caregiving_exchange.asp

Resources Regarding Nonmedical Support

Vet Centers

Call them toll free during normal business hours at 800-905-4675 (Eastern) and 866-496-8838 (Pacific). You can locate a Vet Center near you by going to their website at www.vetcenter.va.gov.

Veterans Service Organizations (VSOs)

A complete listing of all chartered and nonchartered VSOs is available online at www1.va.gov/vso/index.cfm.

Caregiver Support

Call the Administration for Children and Families at 202-401-9215 or visit their site at www.acf.hhs.gov.

Adult Day Care and Adult Social Day

The National Adult Day Services Association can help you find adult day care services that are suitable for your loved one's needs. Visit their site at www.nadsa.org/ or call them at 877-745-1440.

Disability.gov

Disability.gov is the federal government's one-stop website for people with disabilities, their families, employers, veterans and service members, workforce professionals and many others.

The website can be found at www.disability.gov/.

Deployment Health Clinical Center (DHCC)

DHCC at www.pdhealth.mil/hss/smfss.asp offers a list of programs that can assist family members who are caregivers to injured service members.

Family Caregiver Alliance

Family Caregiver Alliance offers a caregiver support group at www.care giver.org/caregiver/jsp/content_node.jsp?nodeid=486. They can also be reached at 415-434-3388 or 800-445-8106.

Their fax is 415-434-3508. You can e-mail them at info@caregiver.org.

Military Aid Societies

- Air Force Aid Society: www.afas.org/ or call them at 800-769-8951.
- Navy Marine Corp Relief Society: www.nmcrs.org/ or call them at 703-696-4904. For a more local number, select the location nearest you from the map located on the webpage at www.nmcrs.org/locations.html.
- Army Emergency Relief: www.aerhq.org/index.asp or call them at 866-878-6378.

National Association of Child Care Resource and Referral Agencies

This site will help you cut the cost of child care if you are the spouse of a service member who is severely injured. Go to www.naccrra.org/MilitaryPrograms/progdesc.php.

National Family Caregivers Association (NFCA)

Call NFCA at 800-896-3650 or visit their site at www.nfcacares.org for resources and information for caregivers.

Transportation Services

To learn about paratransit near you, call Project Action, which maintains a national paratransit database, at 800-659-6428 or 202-347-3066. You can view the database at projectaction.easterseals.com/site/PageServer?pagename = ESPA_rel_links.

National Family Caregivers Support Program

The National Family Caregivers Support Program can be reached at 202-619-0724 and through the Administration on Aging website at www.aoa.gov/.

National Respite Locator Service

To find respite services call 800-773-5433 or visit the National Respite Locator site at www.respitelocator.org/index.htm.

National Women's Health Information Center

Women's health information is available at 800-994-9662.

U.S. National Library of Medicine and the National Institutes of Health

U.S. National Library of Medicine and the National Institutes of Health's website is www.nlm.nih.gov. MedlinePlus provides information for caregivers at www.nlm.nih.gov/medlineplus/caregivers.html. You can e-mail your questions to custserv@nlm.nih.gov. For those who speak Spanish, visit www.nlm.nih.gov/medlineplus/spanish/caregivers.html.

Support Programs

Air Force Wounded Warrior (AFW2) Program

Go to www.woundedwarrior.af.mil, call them at 800-581-9437 between 7 a.m. to 4 p.m. (Central time) or e-mail them at afwounded.warrior@randolph.af.mil. Closed on holidays.

Air Force Survivor Assistance Program

Call 877-USAF-HELP (877-872-3435) any time for support and/or referral to agencies that serve wounded airmen.

America Supports You

A DoD-sponsored site loaded with organizations that want to help severely injured service members and their family. Go to www.ourmilitary.mil/help.shtml for more information.

Army Knowledge Online (AKO)

Army Knowledge Online (AKO) is the U.S. Army's main intranet. It serves registered users to include active duty and retired service personnel and their family members and provides single-sign-on access to over three hundred applications and services. The website is www.us.army.mil.

Army Wounded Warrior Program

You can contact the AW2 Program directly by calling 800-237-1336 between 8 a.m. and 7 p.m. or e-mail them at aw2@conus.army.mil. Visit their website at www.aw2portal.com.

Bar Association

The Bar Association in your community may have a panel that refers callers to lawyers in various specializations. Initial consultations generally include a nominal fee. Visit their website at www.abanet.org/legalservices/findlegalhelp/home.cfm.

GovBenefits.gov

GovBenefits.gov is the official benefits website of the U.S. government, with information on over one thousand benefit and assistance programs. It provides information, fact sheets, and other resources for military personnel, family members, and veterans. The website can be found at www.govbene fits.gov/.

Heroes to Hometown

Learn more about the American Legion program by calling 703-692-2054, or e-mail legion.h2h@itc.dod.mil.

Marine for Life Injured Support

Go to https://wwww.m4l.usmc.mil and click on the purple icon "Injured Marines and Sailors" to get to the site. You can e-mail questions to smbwwropscenter@usmc.mil.

Military Homefront

Military Homefront is the official DoD website for reliable quality-of-life information designed to help troops and their families, leaders, and service providers. The website can be found at www.militaryhomefront.dod.mil/.

Military OneSource/Wounded Warrior Resource Center

Military OneSource is an umbrella service to connect family members to appropriate service-specific and DoD programs and resources that will assist them with their severely injured service member. Military OneSource (including the former Military Severely Injured Center) can be reached at 888-774-1361 or for the Wounded Warrior Resource Center call 800-342-9647. (Both are available 24 hours a day, 7 days a week.) You can also visit their website at www.militaryonesource.com. Click on the Severely Injured tab on the left to get to a page that offers specific information and additional resources.

My Army Benefits

This site produces personalized survivor and retirement benefit reports for active duty soldiers and their family members. It also provides fact sheets on various programs/agencies, including those offered by the various states. The website can be found at myarmybenefits.us.army.mil.

Navy Safe Harbor—Severely Injured Support

The Navy's Safe Harbor program provides personalized assistance to severely injured sailors and their families. Go to their website www.npc .navy.mil/SafeHarbor/. You can e-mail the Safe Harbor program at safe harbor@navy.mil, or can call them at 877-746-8563.

TRICARE

TRICARE Online is the entry point that offers beneficiaries access to available health care services, benefits, and information. The website can be found at www.tricare.mil. Visit their site and take the self-assessment, located at www.tricare.mil/mybenefit/home/MentalHealthAndBehavior/GettingHelp to determine if you could benefit from treatment or evaluation.

Wounded Warrior Project

This project offers programs and services to severely injured service members during the time of active duty to transition to civilian life. It provides direct programs and services to meet their needs. For more information, you may e-mail them at info@woundedwarriorproject.org; call 877-832-6997 or 877-TEAMWWP; or visit their website at www.woundedwarriorproject. org/.

WHERE CAN I FIND ASSISTANCE?

The U.S. Department of Veterans Affairs

The VA is the largest health care system in the United States, with facilities located in every state. We urge you to complete VA Form 10-10EZ to sign up, even if you think you'll never use these services!

Healthcare: 877-222-VETS (8387)
Benefits: 800-827-1000
Website: www.va.gov

VA Medical Centers

The VA services veterans, including the Guard and Reservists. Veterans can receive free services for military-related problems for the first five years following deployment, and copay based on eligibility after that. The VA has many community-based outpatient clinics (CBOCs) located in the community in addition to their medical centers. Find a facility near you. Each medical center has

OEF/OIF Program Manager to help all recent returnees
Health and Mental Health Services
Women Veterans Program Manager
Social Work Services
VA Chaplain

Vet Centers

Vet Centers assist veterans and their families in making a successful postwar adjustment, offering

Readjustment counseling (including PTSD treatment)
Marriage and family, benefits, bereavement, alcohol and drug counseling
Job services and help obtaining services at the VA and community agencies

There are no copayments or charges for Vet Center services, and services are completely confidential. The Readjustment Counseling Service can be reached by calling toll-free 800-905-4675, or visiting their website at www.va .gov/rcs.

Other Resources

Military OneSource

This resource helps military members, veterans, and families deal with life issues 24/7. Service members and family members can call in and speak to a master's level consultant who can answer almost any question, no matter how big or small.

Toll-free (in the U.S.): 800-342-9647
Toll-free (outside the U.S.): (country access code) 800-342-9647 (dial all 11 numbers)
International toll-free: 800-464-8107
Website: www.militaryonesource.com/ (user id: military; password: one-source)

Veterans Service Organizations (VSOs)

VSOs can help you to complete necessary paperwork and to navigate the VA system. They include organizations such as the American Legion, the VFW, AMVETS, Disabled American Veterans (DAV), and more. The Directory of Veterans Service Organizations can be accessed at www1.va.gov/vso/index.cfm?template = view. Additional information about local VSOs is listed at the end of this chapter.

State Resources

All states have a variety of programs and resources for veterans and their families. Most states have an information and referral line, such as dialing 2-1-1 (visit 211.org to see what your state offers). Or call your local

Agency or Department of Health and or Human Services
State's Office of Veterans Affairs (NASDVA)
Veteran representatives in the offices of legislative officials

Employer Support of the Guard and Reserves (ESGR)

ESGR provides assistance with issues between service members and employers. Contact them toll-free (in the U.S.) at 800-336-4590, or by visiting their website at www.esgr.org.

Veterans Transition Assistance Representative

The Transition Assistance Program is a collaboration of DoD, VA, and the Department of Labor to help with transition from military to civilian life. Their website is www.transitionassistanceprogram.com/register.tpp.

Chaplains and Other Religious Leaders

Every VA Medical Center and military establishment has a chaplain on staff who can provide you assistance. All information exchanges with a chaplain are confidential.

Local Family Assistance Centers

The National Guard Bureau provides family assistance in every state for all military family members, no matter the branch of service. Visit www.guardfamily.org/Public/Application/ResourceFinderSearch.aspx and click on your state to find locations near you, or call 703-607-5414.

Employment and Financial Services
Additional assistance may be available through these resources:

U.S. Department of Labor
Vet Success
Deployment Support Resources

Veterans Service Organizations
The below listing is alphabetical by name of the organization.

African American Post Traumatic Stress Disorder Association
Lakewood, WA, 253-589-0766, www.aaptsdassn.org

Air Force Sergeants Association
Suitland, MD, 301-899-3500, www.hqafsa.org

American Ex-Prisoners of War
Arlington, TX, 817-649-2979, www.axpow.org

American GI Forum of the United States
Denver, CO, 303-458-1700, www.agif.us

American Gold Star Mothers, Inc
Washington, DC, 202-265-0991, www.goldstarmoms.com

American Legion
Indianapolis, IN, 317-630-1200, www.legion.org

American War Mothers
Washington, DC, 202-362-0090, www.americanwarmoms.org

AMVETS
Lanham, MD, 301-459-9600, www.amvets.org

Armed Forces Service Corp.
Arlington, VA, 703-379-9311, www.afsc-usa.com

Army and Navy Union, USA, Inc.
Niles, OH, 330-307-7049, www.armynavy.net

Blinded Veterans Association
Washington, DC, 202-371-8880, www.bva.org

Blue Star Mothers of America, Inc.
Montpelier, VA, 505-352-2941 (fax), www.bluestarmothers.org

Catholic War Veterans
Alexandria, VA, 703-549-3622, www.cwv.org

Congressional Medal of Honor Society of the United States of America
Mt. Pleasant, SC, 843-884-8862, www.cmohs.org

Disabled American Veterans
Cold Spring, KY, 859-441-7300, www.dav.org

Fleet Reserve Association
Alexandria, VA, 800-372-1924, www.fra.org

Gold Star Wives of America, Inc.
Birmingham, AL, 703-351-6246, www.goldstarwives.org

Italian American War Veterans of the USA
Youngstown, OH, 772-581-8050, www.ITAMVETS.org

Jewish War Veterans of the USA
Washington, DC, 202-265-6280, www.jwv.org

Legion of Valor of the USA, Inc.
Santa Barbara, CA, 805-692-2244, www.legionofvalor.com

Marine Corps League
Fairfax, VA, 703-207-9588/99, www.mcleague.org

Military Chaplains Association of the United States of America
Arlington, VA, 703-533-5890, www.mca-usa.org

Military Order of the Purple Heart of the USA, Inc.
Springfield, VA, 703-354-2140, www.purpleheart.org

Military Order of the World Wars
Alexandria, VA, 703-683-4911, www.militaryorder.net

National Amputation Foundation, Inc.
Malverne, NY, 516-887-3600, www.nationalamputation.org

National Association for Black Veterans, Inc.
Milwaukee, WI, 800-842-4597, www.nabvets.com

National Association of County Veterans Service Officers, Inc.
Arlington, VA, 910-592-2862, www.nacvso.org

National Association of State Directors of Veterans Affairs
Madison, WI, 608-266-1311, www.nasdva.com

National Veterans Legal Services Program
Washington, DC, 202-265-8305, www.nvlsp.org

Navy Club of the United States of America
Lafayette, IN, 800-628-7265, www.navyclubusa.org

Navy Mutual Aid Association
Arlington, VA, 571-481-2324, www.navymutual.org

Non Commissioned Officers Association
San Antonio, TX, 210-653-6161, www.ncoausa.org

Paralyzed Veterans of America
Washington, DC, 202-872-1300, www.pva.org

Polish Legion of American Veterans, USA
Washington, DC, 727-848-7826, www.plav.org

Swords to Plowshares: Veterans Rights Organization
San Francisco, CA, 415-252-4788, www.swords-to-plowshares.org

The Retired Enlisted Association
Aurora, CO, 800-338-9337, www.trea.org

United Spinal Association
Jackson Heights, NY, 718-803-3782, www.unitedspinal.org

Veterans Assistance Foundation, Inc.
Newburg, WI, 262-692-6333, www.veteransassistance.org

Veterans of Foreign Wars of the United Sates
Kansas City, MO, 816-756-3390, www.vfw.org

Veterans of the Vietnam War, Inc./Veterans Coalition
Pittston, PA, 570-603-9740, www.vvnw.org

Women's Army Corps Veterans Association
Fort McClellan, AL, 256-820-6824, www.armywomen.org

Glossary

activities of daily living (ADL). The inability to carry out activities of daily living means the inability to independently perform at least two of the six following functions:

1. Bathing
2. Continence
3. Dressing
4. Eating
5. Toileting
6. Transferring in or out of a bed or chair with or without equipment

Air Force Assistance Fund (AFAF). An aid organization that serves the Air Force.

Air Force Board of Correction of Military Records (AFBCMR). The final appeal authority for a member of the U.S. Air Force who disagrees with the findings or disposition determination of a formal PEB that has been upheld by the SAFPC.

Air Force Wounded Warrior (AFW2) Program. The AFW2 Program provides personalized care and services to any airman ill or injured in support of OEF and OIF. Advocates for services on an airman's behalf, they ensure airmen have professional support and follow-up for no less than five years after separation or retirement.

America Supports You (ASY). America Supports You is a website that connects people, organizations, and companies to hundreds of groups that offer a variety of support to the military community.

Americans with Disabilities Act (ADA). Signed into law in 1990, the Americans with Disabilities Act is a civil rights law that, in many cases, prohibits discrimination based on disability.

America's Job Bank. America's Job Bank is a service of the Department of Labor and the individual state employment services.

Army Board for the Correction of Military Records (ABCMR). The final appeal authority for a member of the U.S. Army who disagrees with the findings or disposition determination of a formal PEB that has been upheld by the USAPDA.

Army Career and Alumni Program (ACAP). ACAP is a world-class transition and job assistance services program for soldiers and civilian employees and their family members.

Army Emergency Relief (AER). An aid organization that serves the Army.

Army Knowledge Online (AKO). AKO is the U.S. Army's main intranet. It serves registered users to include active duty and retired service personnel and their family members, and provides single-sign-on access to over three hundred applications and services.

Army Wounded Warrior Program (AW2). The program's mission is to provide personalized support for severely injured soldiers, no matter where they are located or how long their recovery takes.

Basic Allowance for Subsistence (BAS). A payment to members for food. Members who are hospitalized continue receiving BAS during the hospitalization.

Board for Correction of Naval Records (BCNR). The final appeal authority for a member of the U.S. Navy or U.S. Marine Corps who disagrees with the findings or disposition determination of a formal PEB that has been upheld by the DIRSECNAVCORB.

casual pay. Army term for an advance on a member's end-of-month paycheck. This payment will be automatically deducted during subsequent pay periods until paid back.

Centers for Disease Control and Prevention (CDC). The CDC is a government agency with the mission of promoting health and quality of life by preventing and controlling disease, injury, and disability. It is performing Vietnam veteran, Gulf War veteran, and Force Health Protections studies to evaluate the conditions of veterans as well as the care they receive.

civilian legal counsel. Members may hire, with their own funds, a civilian lawyer to represent them during formal PEB hearings.

Combat Related Injury and Rehabilitation Pay (CIP). A monthly payment for members who were evacuated from a combat zone due to an injury. This payment was replaced by PAC, but some members who were wounded before PAC was established may be eligible for back payment of the allowance.

Combat-Related Special Compensation (CRSC). A monthly compensation that is intended to replace some or all of members' retired pay that is withheld due to receipt of VA compensation.

Combat Zone Tax Exclusion (CZTE). A policy that exempts a member from paying federal taxes while serving in an area designated as a combat zone.

combat/operational stress injuries (COSI). Changes in mental functioning or behavior due to the challenges of combat and its aftermath, or changes in mental functioning or behavior due to the challenges of military operations other than combat.

combined rating. The total percentage of disability for a member with more than one disability. This is not determined by adding percentages of disability for each condition. The formula for determining a combined rating can be found in Section 4.25 (table 1) of Title 38 of the Code of Federal Regulations.

community based health care organization (CBHCO). If you are a member of the Army National Guard and Army Reserve and require only outpatient care, you may request transfer to a CBHCO. This program allows you to live at home, receive outpatient care, and perform military duties at a local military organization such as an armory or recruiting station. You cannot work at a civilian job while you are attached to a CBHCO.

Computer/Electronic Accommodations Program (CAP). CAP is the federal government's centrally funded accommodation program.

Concurrent Retirement and Disability Payments (CRDP). A program that restores retired pay on a graduated ten-year schedule for retirees with a 50 to 90 percent VA-rated disability.

Continued Health Care Benefit Program (CHCBP). The CHCBP is similar to but is not TRICARE. It offers temporary transitional health coverage and must be purchased within thirty days after your TRICARE eligibility ends. Benefits under CHCBP are virtually the same as those under TRS, and your coverage will start the day after your separation.

DD Form 214—Certificate of Release or Discharge from Active Duty. The Report of Separation contains information normally needed to verify military service for benefits, retirement, employment, and membership in veterans' organizations.

DD Form 2586—Verification of Military Experience and Training. The DD

Form 2586 is created from a service member's automated records on file. It lists military job experience and training history, recommended college credit information, and civilian-equivalent job titles. This document is designed to help the member apply for jobs, but it is not a resume.

DD Form 2648 Pre-separation Counseling Checklist. A form used by the DoD that helps Transition Assistance Program employees assist members in transitioning out of the military and into civilian life.

Department of Veterans Affairs (VA). The federal agency responsible for providing a broad range of programs and services to service members and veterans as required by Title 38 of the U.S. Code.

Director, Secretary of the Navy Council of Review Boards (DIRSECNAVC-ORB). The governing body for the U.S. Navy overseeing the DES process for the service. A sailor or marine may appeal a PEB finding with the DIRSEC-NAVCORB, which has the authority to uphold the PEB findings, issue revised findings, or send the case back to the PEB for another review.

Disability Evaluation System (DES). A system or process of the U.S. government for evaluating the nature and extent of disabilities affecting members of the armed forces; it includes medical/psychological evaluations, physical evaluations, counseling of members, and mechanisms for the final disposition of disability determinations.

Disability Evaluation System (DES) Pilot. A joint DoD-VA Disability Evaluation System Pilot was begun in the National Capital Region in November 2007 to improve the timeliness, effectiveness, and transparency of the DES review process. Under the pilot, VA performs one medical exam and rates a member's disabilities. This examination and rating is used by the PEB to determine fitness for duty and disposition, and by VA to determine VA disability compensation.

disability retirement pay. The monthly allowance paid to members who are placed on the TDRL or PDRL. The formula for determining the amount of disability retirement pay is found in chapter 9.

Disabled Transition Assistance Program (DTAP). DTAP works with members who may be released because of a disability or who believe they have a disability qualifying them for VA's Vocational Rehabilitation and Employment Program (VR&E). The goal of DTAP is to encourage and assist potentially eligible service members in making an informed decision about VA's VR&E program. It is also intended to quickly deliver vocational rehabilitation services to eligible service members by assisting them in filing an application for vocational rehabilitation benefits.

Disabled Veterans Outreach Program (DVOP) Specialists. A Department of Labor employee trained to help veterans make the important adjustment to the civilian job market.

DoD Job Search. A website that is a part of the America's Job Bank service designed solely for service members.

DoD Suicide Prevention and Risk Reduction Committee's (SPARRC) Preventing Suicide Network. The DoD SPARRC Preventing Suicide Network is a resource center aimed at providing authoritative and problem-specific information about suicide prevention.

efficiency. Efficiency is the measure of a member's total health minus his or her disability. A member with a 60 percent disability has only 40 percent of his or her total health that is not impacted by the disability.

Family and Medical Leave Act (FMLA). The federal law that provides unpaid leave and job protection to those who have family members with medical conditions that require their presence. The Fiscal Year 2008 National Defense Authorization Act authorized the expansion of the FMLA to support families of recovering service members.

Family Liaison Officer (FLO). An Air Force employee appointed to every airman with a combat-related injury to assist in providing support to the recovering airman's family.

Family Separation Allowance (FSA). Pay a member receives if he or she has dependents and is away from his or her permanent duty station for more than thirty days for temporary duty or on a temporary change of station, to include a deployment.

fit/unfit. Finding of the PEB. Fitness or unfitness is solely determined by the ability of the member to perform the duties of his or her office, grade, rank, or rating because of disease or injury.

formal Physical Evaluation Board (PEB). If a member disagrees with the informal PEB findings or disposition, he or she may request a formal PEB, appear before the board in person, obtain military or civilian legal counsel to represent him or her, call witnesses, present evidence, and present testimony on his or her own behalf.

GL-2005.261—Traumatic Injury Protection Payment. The form used to request insurance payment for service-connected traumatic injury or loss from service in OIF/OEF.

Hardship Duty Pay Location (HDP-L). Pay a member receives while serving in a location that the Secretary of Defense identifies as a hardship duty location.

Health and Human Services (HHS). HHS is the principal agency for protecting the health of all Americans and providing essential human services, especially for those who are least able to help themselves.

Health Resources and Service Administration (HRSA). HRSA is the primary federal agency for improving access to health care services for people who are uninsured, isolated, or medically vulnerable.

hemiplegia. Paralysis affecting only one side of the body.

hospitalized. For the purposes of some pay entitlements, members are considered hospitalized if they were admitted as an inpatient or were receiving extensive rehabilitation as an outpatient while living in quarters affiliated with the military health care system.

Hostile Fire Pay/Imminent Danger Pay (HFP/IDP). Pay a member receives while serving in an area the president identifies as placing him or her in imminent danger or that he or she may come under hostile fire.

Individual Transition Plan (ITP). The ITP is a framework a member can use to fulfill realistic career goals based upon his or her unique skills, knowledge, experience, and abilities. The ITP identifies actions and activities associated with a member's transition.

informal Physical Evaluation Board. The initial meeting of a PEB to determine a disposition of the member's medical case. The member will not be present at the informal PEB. The informal PEB will determine fit/unfit and the member's disposition based on the member's case file. The PEBLO counsels the member on the findings of the informal PEB and provide options for appeal of those findings.

Invitational Travel Authorizations (ITAs), Invitational Travel Orders (ITOs), or Emergency Family Member Travel (EFMT). Military travel orders that allow a recovering service member's family to travel and stay with him or her during treatment and recovery after suffering a wound, illness, or injury.

Job Accommodation Network (JAN). A free service from the Department of Labor's Office of Disability Employment Policy that provides personalized worksite accommodations, information regarding the ADA and other disability-related information, and information about self-employment.

local veterans employment representative (LVER). A Department of Labor employee trained to help veterans make the important adjustment to the civilian job market.

Medical Evaluation Board (MEB). A board, generally comprising medical officers, that determines if a member meets medical retention standards for his or her service. The board may recommend a return to duty or send the member's case to a Physical Evaluation Board.

MedlinePlus. MedlinePlus is a service of the U.S. National Library of Medicine and the National Institutes of Health that provides resources regarding all aspects of veterans' health including recent news, treatments, rehabilitation and recovery programs, condition-specific information, financial issues, as well as ongoing clinical trials and research.

mild traumatic brain injury (mTBI). Mild traumatic brain injury (concussion) is caused by blunt trauma to the head or acceleration/deceleration forces jogging the brain within the skull, which may or may not produce a period of unconsciousness. Mild TBI is defined as an injury to the brain as a result of any period of observed or self-reported confusion, disorientation, or impaired consciousness; dysfunction of memory around the time of injury (amnesia); or loss of consciousness lasting less than thirty minutes. No other obvious neurological deficits or intracranial complications (e.g., hematoma/blood clot) should be found, and normal computed tomography (CT) findings should be present.

Military Severely Injured Center (MSIC). A DoD call-in support program that provides information regarding medical care and rehabilitation; education, training, and job placement; personal mobility and functioning; accommodations; counseling; and financial resources.

minority opinion. When a member of the PEB disagrees with the findings of the board, he or she will write a minority opinion outlining the areas of disagreement that becomes part of the board findings.

Montgomery G.I. Bill (MGIB). The MGIB provides up to thirty-six months of education benefits to eligible veterans for college, technical, or vocational courses; correspondence courses; apprenticeship/job training; flight training; high-tech training; licensing and certification tests; entrepreneurship training; and certain entrance examinations.

Montgomery G.I. Bill—Selected Reserve (MGIB-SR). The MGIB-SR program may be available to you if you are a member of the Selected Reserve. The Selected Reserve includes the Army Reserve, Navy Reserve, Air Force Reserve, Marine Corps Reserve, and Coast Guard Reserve, and the Army National Guard and the Air National Guard. You may use this education assistance program for degree programs, certificate or correspondence courses, cooperative training, independent study programs, apprenticeship/on-the-job training, and vocational flight training programs.

National Association for People of Color Against Suicide (NOPCAS). NOPCAS is a nonprofit organization with the goal of stopping suicide in minority communities.

National Association of Child Care Resource and Referral Agencies (NACCRRA). NACCRRA is an organization through which a service member can get assistance to find and pay for safe, licensed child care services for a period of six months during his or her recuperation.

National Capital Region (NCR). Washington, D.C., and the surrounding areas.

National Defense Authorization Act for Fiscal Year 2008 (NDAA). Public Law 110-181 that authorizes expenditures and provides guidance for the federal government concerning national defense. In the Fiscal Year 2008 version, a large section was devoted to wounded warrior issues.

National Institute of Diabetes, Digestive and Kidney Diseases (NIDDK). NIDDK supports twenty-two research projects related to veterans of military service.

National Institute of Mental Health (NIMH). NIMH conducts projects on trauma and post-traumatic stress disorder that involve veteran populations.

National Institute on Deafness and Other Communicative Disorders (NIDCD). The NIDCD studies the molecular mechanisms that cause the loss of hearing from exposure to loud noise.

National Institute on Dental and Craniofacial Research (NIDCR). The NIDCR conducts ongoing research in tissue engineering and regeneration for wounds to the head and face.

National Strategy for Suicide Prevention (NSSP). The NSSP is a collaborative effort between SAMSHA, CDC, NIH, HRSA, and HHS and provides facts about suicide, recent publications, and resources designed to spread knowledge of the seriousness of suicides.

Navy Marine Corps Relief Society (NMCRS). An aid organization that serves the Navy and Marine Corps.

Navy Safe Harbor. The Navy Safe Harbor program provides personalized assistance to severely injured sailors and their families.

ombudsman. An ombudsman is assigned to or near a major military facility or VA medical facility to further assist in the transition by helping service members connect with local agencies and community groups.

Operation Enduring Freedom (OEF). OEF includes casualties that occurred

In and Around Afghanistan: in Afghanistan, Pakistan, and Uzbekistan.
Other Locations: in Guantanamo Bay (Cuba), Djibouti, Eritrea, Ethiopia,
Jordan, Kenya, Kyrgyzstan, Philippines, Seychelles, Sudan, Tajikistan,
Turkey, and Yemen.

Operation Iraqi Freedom (OIF). OIF includes casualties that occurred on or
after March 19, 2003, in the Arabian Sea, Bahrain, Gulf of Aden, Gulf of
Oman, Iraq, Kuwait, Oman, Persian Gulf, Qatar, Red Sea, Saudi Arabia, and
United Arab Emirates. Prior to March 19, 2003, casualties in these countries
were considered OEF.

paraplegia. Complete paralysis of the lower half of the body, including both
legs, usually caused by damage to the spinal cord.

partial pay. Air Force term for an advance on a member's end-of-month paycheck. This payment will be automatically deducted during subsequent pay
periods until paid back.

Patient Administration Team (PAT). A nonmedical care organization that as-
sists members of the military in issues related to their hospitalization and
recovery.

Pay and Allowance Continuation (PAC). A new policy allowing members
evacuated from a combat zone to continue receiving all combat pay and allowances they received prior to the injury for the first year they are hospitalized.

per diem. A daily allowance paid to a person on military travel orders to
cover food, lodging, and incidentals. In cases where lodging or food is provided by the government, this payment will only be for the $3.50 incidental
rate.

Permanent Disabled Retirement List (PDRL). The PEB disposition finding for
a member who has one or more service unfitting condition(s) with a combined rating of 30 percent or higher, was incurred in the line of duty, and is
considered stable. This disposition also covers members who have served
twenty or more years, have one or more service unfitting condition(s) with a
combined rating of 20 percent or less, was incurred in the line of duty, and
are considered stable.

Personnel Service Detachment (PSD). A military personnel office that will
assist members and their families with pay and personnel problems.

Physical Evaluation Board (PEB). A board, generally comprising a senior line officer, senior personnel officer, and senior medical officer, that determines if a member is fit or unfit for continued service. This board may recommend a return to duty, separation with or without benefits, or medical retirement (temporary or permanent).

Physical Evaluation Board Disposition. The findings of a PEB on a member's medical case. Member can be found fit and returned to duty, found unfit and separated with or without benefits, or medically retired on either the Permanent or Temporary Disability Retirement List.

Physical Evaluation Board Liaison Officer (PEBLO). The person assigned to assist the service member through the DES process. Duties include counseling the member on the process as well as building the case file used by the PEB to determine fitness for duty.

Post-9/11 G.I. Bill. Post-9/11 G.I. Bill is a new benefit providing educational assistance to individuals who have served on active duty on or after September 11, 2001. It provides additional monetary benefits for members, including a housing and book allowance, and is limited by the cost of the highest public school tuition costs in the state, where the member resides, rather than a set cap like in the Montgomery G.I. Bill. It also allows for transfer of benefits to family members in certain instances.

post-traumatic stress disorder (PTSD). A traumatic stress injury that fails to heal such that the symptoms and behaviors it causes remain significantly troubling or disabling beyond thirty days after their onset.

Project Action. Project Action maintains a national paratransit database.

quadriplegia. Paralysis of all four limbs.

REALifelines. A Department of Labor program to help injured veterans return to fulfilling, productive civilian lives using federal, state, and local-level efforts to create a network of resources that focus on veteran well-being and job-placement assistance.

Recovery Coordinator. A person assigned to make sure your needs are being met by the right person in the right place and on time.

Recovery Plan. The Recovery Coordinator prepares a Recovery Plan that lays out the path for you to meet personal and professional goals.

respite care. Respite care includes adult day care and home care services, as well as overnight stays in a facility, and can be provided a few hours a week or for a weekend.

return to duty. The PEB disposition finding for a member who does not have a service unfitting condition.

Savings Deposit Program (SDP). Members deployed to combat zones may put up to $10,000 of their pay in this program and earn 10 percent interest on the money deposited.

Secretary of the Air Force Personnel Council (SAFPC). Organization that can uphold a PEB finding, revise the findings of a PEB, or return the case to the PEB for further review. Airmen may present a written rebuttal to the SAFPC if they disagree with the PEB findings.

separate with severance pay. The PEB disposition finding for a member who has a service unfitting condition, but whose combined rating is 20 percent or less.

separate without benefits. The PEB disposition finding for a member who has a service unfitting condition, but whose condition is not found to be in the line of duty, or is found to have existed before entry into service and not aggravated by service.

Servicemembers' Group Life Insurance (SGLI). SGLI is a program of low-cost group life insurance for service members on active duty, ready reservists, members of the National Guard, members of the Commissioned Corps of the National Oceanic and Atmospheric Administration and the Public Health Service, cadets and midshipmen of the four service academies, and members of the Reserve Officer Training Corps.

severance pay. A one-time, lump-sum payment for members separated from the military for medical reasons, but who receive a combined rating of 20 percent or less for unfitting conditions. The formula for determining the amount of service pay a member will receive is found in chapter 9.

SGLV 8714—Veterans Group Life Insurance (VGLI). The form used to convert SGLI to VGLI.

SGLV 8715—SGLI Disability Extension. The form used to request an extension of the SGLI coverage for two years from date of discharge from the military for those who are totally disabled.

Small Business Administration (SBA) loans. Business loans are available to veterans through programs of the SBA. In addition, SBA offers loans specifically to Vietnam-era and disabled veterans.

Social Security Administration (SSA). The SSA is the government agency that is charged with ensuring the economic security of Americans. While you work you pay taxes into the Social Security system, and when you retire or become disabled, you, your spouse, and your dependent children receive monthly benefits that are based on your reported earnings. Also, your survivors can collect benefits if you die.

Social Security Disability Insurance Program (SSDI). SSDI pays benefits to you and certain members of your family if you are "insured," meaning that you worked long enough and paid Social Security taxes.

special pay. Navy/Marine Corps term for an advance on a member's end-of-month paycheck. This payment will be automatically deducted during subsequent pay periods until paid back.

stable. A condition that, in the doctor's opinion, is unlikely to improve to the point at which a member can return to duty.

Substance Abuse and Mental Health Services Administration (SAMHSA). SAMHSA is an agency within the DHHS that focuses on building resilience and facilitating recovery for people with or at risk for mental or substance use disorders.

Suicide Awareness Voices of Education (SAVE). SAVE is a nonprofit organization with the goal of preventing suicide through public awareness and education, reducing stigma, and serving as a resource for those touched by suicide.

Supplemental Security Income (SSI). SSI is a federal income supplement program funded by general tax revenues (not Social Security taxes). It is designed to help aged, blind, and disabled people who have little or no income and provides cash to meet basic needs for food, clothing, and shelter.

Temporary Disability Retirement List (TDRL). The PEB disposition finding for a member who has one or more service unfitting condition(s) with a combined rating of 30 percent or higher, was incurred in the line of duty, and is not considered stable.

Transition Assistance Program (TAP). TAP is a program designed to ease the transition from military service to the civilian workforce and community.

traumatic brain injury (TBI). Traumatic brain injury is a neurological injury with possible physical, cognitive, behavioral, and emotional symptoms. Like all injuries, TBI is most appropriately and accurately diagnosed as soon as possible after the injury. TBI is not a mental health condition. The range of TBI includes mild, moderate, severe, and penetrating. Well after the injury event, service personnel may have residual symptoms from a TBI and new or emerging PTSD symptoms. If the TBI has not been previously identified or documented, an accurate description of the traumatic events in theater usually allows a well-trained clinician to make a distinction between TBI and PTSD or other mental health conditions.

traumatic event. A qualifying traumatic injury is an injury or loss caused by application of external force or violence (a traumatic event) *or* a condition whose cause can be directly linked to a traumatic event.

traumatic injury. Traumatic injury is derived by external force or violence or a condition that can be linked to a traumatic event.

Traumatic Servicemembers' Group Life Insurance (TSGLI). An insurance program related to the Servicemembers' Group Life Insurance that pays a member who has suffered a severe loss, such as a leg or arm amputation.

TRICARE. The military medical health care system.

TRICARE Dental Program (TDP). The dental insurance coverage offered to those who are TRICARE eligible.

TRICARE Online. TRICARE Online is the entry point that offers beneficiaries access to available health care services, benefits, and information.

TRICARE Reserve Select (TRS). TRS is a premium-based plan that you purchase. You may receive care from any TRICARE-authorized provider without a referral. Referrals are not required, but some medical services will require prior authorization. For information or assistance with qualifying for and purchasing TRS, check the TRICARE website.

Troops to Teachers (TTT). The TTT program is funded and overseen by the Department of Education and operated by the DoD. The TTT program helps recruit quality teachers for schools that serve students from low-income families throughout America.

U.S. Air Force Physical Disability Division. Processing agency for all formal and informal PEB cases in the U.S. Air Force. This organization reviews all PEB findings and dispositions, referring those it feels need further review to the Secretary of the Air Force Personnel Council.

U.S. Army Physical Disability Agency (USAPDA). The governing body for the U.S. Army overseeing the DES process for the service. All PEB findings are sent to the USAPDA, and 20 percent of the cases are randomly reviewed for quality assurance purposes. Any case with a minority opinion will be automatically reviewed. Soldiers may appeal a PEB finding with the USAPDA, which has the authority to uphold the PEB findings, issue revised findings, or send the case back to the PEB for another review.

U.S. Public Health Service (USPHS). "Healthier Vets," the Surgeon General's joint DHHS-VA initiative, is designed to help veterans and their families remain physically active after they have separated from the military.

unemployment compensation for ex-service members. Service members separating from active duty may qualify for unemployment compensation if they are unable to find a new job.

VA Form 10-8678—Clothing Allowance. The form used to apply for a clothing allowance if a service-connected disability requiring a prosthetic device or orthopedic appliance (such as a wheelchair) leads to damage to a veteran's clothes.

VA Form 21-4502—Vehicle Purchase and Adaptation. The form used to apply for a one-time grant toward the purchase of a vehicle with adaptive equipment approved by VA for a veteran or service member with certain disabilities.

VA Form 21-526—Compensation and Pension. The form used to request VA provide service-related disability compensation, or a pension for those who are wartime veterans with non-service-connected disabilities.

VA Form 21-8940—Increased Compensation Based on Unemployability. The form used to request compensation based on an inability to work due to total disability from service-connected disability(s).

VA Form 22-1990—VA Education Benefits. The form used to apply for multiple education benefits, including the Montgomery G.I. Bill Educational Assistance Program; Montgomery G.I. Bill Selected Reserve Educational Assistance Program; Reserve Educational Assistance Program; Post-Vietnam Era Veterans Educational Assistance Program; National Call to Serve Program; and the Transfer of Entitlement Program.

VA Form 22-5490—Survivors' and Dependents' Educational Assistance. The form used to apply for educational assistance to a spouse or child if the member is permanently and totally disabled as a result of a service-connected disability, dies of a service-connected disability, or while rated permanently and totally disabled, or is missing in action or a prisoner of war.

VA Form 26-4555—Housing Adaptation. The form used to apply for grants for constructing an adapted home or modifying an existing home to meet a disabled veteran/service member's needs.

VA Form 28-1900—Disabled Veterans Application for Vocational Rehabilitation. The form used to apply for vocational rehabilitation and employment benefits.

VA Form 28-8832—Application for Counseling. The form used to apply for vocational and educational counseling

VA Form 29-0188—Application for Supplemental Service-Disabled Veterans (RH) Life Insurance. The form used to apply for Supplemental Service-Disabled Veterans Insurance.

VA Form 29-357—Claim for Disability Insurance Benefits. The form used to apply for waiver of premiums on a Service-Disabled Veterans Insurance policy.

VA Form 29-4364—Application for Service-Disabled Veterans Life Insurance. The form used to apply for Service-Disabled Veterans Insurance (S-DVI).

VA Form 29-8636—Veterans Mortgage Life Insurance Statement. The form used to apply for Veterans Mortgage Life Insurance (VMLI).

VA Schedule for Rating Disabilities (VASRD). The document used to determine the severity of a member's disability expressed as a percentage of disability.

Vet Center Program. Vet Centers, run by VA, provide free individual, group, and family counseling to all veterans who served in any combat zone.

Veterans Educational Assistance Program (VEAP). VEAP is available if you elected to make contributions from your military pay to participate in this education benefit program. You may use these benefits for degree, certificate, correspondence, apprenticeship/on-the-job training programs, and vocational flight training programs. In certain circumstances, remedial, deficiency, and refresher training may also be available. Benefit entitlement is one to thirty-six months depending on the number of monthly contributions. You have ten years from your release from active duty to use VEAP benefits. If there is entitlement not used after the ten-year period, your portion remaining in the fund will be automatically refunded.

Veterans Preference (federal hiring). Veterans who are disabled, served on active duty in the military during certain specified time periods, or in military campaigns, are entitled to preference over others in hiring for virtually all federal government jobs.

Veterans Upward Bound (VUB) program. The VUB program is a free Department of Education program designed to help eligible U.S. military veterans refresh their academic skills so that they can successfully complete the postsecondary school of their choosing.

Veterans Service Organization (VSO). Organizations that are chartered by

Congress and/or recognized by VA for claims representation for today's returning service members, veterans, and their families.

Vocational Rehabilitation and Employment (VR&E). VR&E delivers timely and effective vocational rehabilitation services to veterans with service-connected disabilities and to certain service members awaiting discharge due to a medical condition.

Wounded Warrior Pay Management Team (WWPMT). Highly trained finance experts who the Defense Finance and Accounting Service have prepared to deal with the complex issues surrounding pay and allowances for recovering service members.

Wounded Warrior Project (WWP). A project offering programs and services to severely injured members during the time of active duty through transition to civilian life.

Wounded Warrior Regiment/Marine for Life Injured Support. The program is to "provide information, advocacy and assistance to injured Marines, Sailors injured while serving with Marines, and their families, in order to minimize the difficulties and worries they face as they navigate the stressful and confusing process."

References

Beck, A.T., & Steer, R.A. (2000). Beck Depression Inventory. In Task Force for the Handbook of Psychiatric Measures (Ed.), *Handbook of psychiatric measures* (pp. 519–522). Washington, DC: American Psychiatric Association.

Benedek, D.M., Ursano, R.J., Holloway, H.C., Norwood, A.E., Grieger, T.A., Engel, C.C., et al. (2001). Military and disaster psychiatry. In N.J. Smelser & P.B. Baltes (Eds.), *International encyclopedia of the social and behavioral sciences*, vol. 14 (pp. 9850–9857). Oxford, England: Elsevier Science.

Bien, T. H., Miller, W. R., & Tonigan, J. S. (1993). Brief interventions for alcohol problems: a review. *Addiction, 88*, 315–335.

Briere, J. (1997). *Psychological assessment of adult posttraumatic states*. Washington, DC: American Psychological Association.

Brom, D., Kleber, R.J., & Hofman, M.C. (1993). Victims of traffic accidents: Incidence and prevention of post-traumatic stress disorder. *Journal of Clinical Psychology, 49*, 131–140.

Bryant, R.A., Guthrie, R.M., & Moulds, M.L. (2001). Hypnotizability in acute stress disorder. *American Journal of Psychiatry, 158*, 600–604.

Bryant, R.A., & Harvey, A.G. (2000). *Acute stress disorder: A handbook of theory, assessment, and treatment*. Washington, D.C.: American Psychological Association

Bryant, R. A., Harvey, A. G., Dang, S. T., Sackville, T., & Basten, C. (1998). Treatment of acute stress disorder: A comparison of cognitive-behavioral therapy and supportive counseling. *Journal of Consulting and Clinical Psychology, 66*, 862–866.

Bryant, R. A., Sackville, T., Dang, S. T., Moulds, M., & Guthrie, R. (1999). Treating acute stress disorder: An evaluation of cognitive behavior therapy and supportive counseling techniques. *American Journal of Psychiatry, 156*, 1780–1786.

Buss, A.H., & Durkee, A. (1957). An inventory for assessing different kinds of hostility. *Journal of Counseling Psychology, 21*, 343–349.

Buss, A.H., & Perry, M. (1992). The Aggression Questionnaire. *Journal of Personality and Social Psychology, 63*, 452–459.

Carlson, E.B. (November, 2002). *Challenges to assessing traumatic stress histories in complex trauma survivors.* Paper presented at the Annual meeting of the International Society for Traumatic Stress Studies, Baltimore, MD.

Carlson, E.B. (1997). *Trauma assessments: A clinician's guide.* New York: Guilford Press.

Carlson, E.B., & Waelde, L. (November, 2000). *Preliminary psychometric properties of the Trauma Related Dissociation Scale.* Paper presented at the Annual Meeting of the International Society for Traumatic Stress Studies, San Antonio, TX.

Chemtob, C.M., Novaco, R.W., Hamada, R.S., Gross, D.M., & Smith, G. (1997). Anger regulation deficits in combat-related posttraumatic stress disorder. *Journal of Traumatic Stress, 10,* 17–36.

Dawson, D. (2000). US low risk drinking guidelines: An examination of four alternatives. *Alcoholism Clinical and Experimental Research, 24,* 1820–1829.

DiGiovanni, C., Jr. (1999). Domestic terrorism with chemical or biological agents: Psychiatric aspects. *American Journal of Psychiatry, 156,* 1500–1505.

Dunning, C. M. (1996). From citizen to soldier: Mobilization of reservists. In R. J. Ursano & A. E. Norwood (Eds.), *Emotional aftermath of the Persian Gulf War: Veterans, families, communities, and nations* (pp. 197–225). Washington, DC: American Psychiatric Press.

Elsayed, N.M. (1997). Toxicology of blast overpressure. *Toxicology. 121*(1):1–15.

Foa, E. B., Keane, T. M., & Friedman, M. J. (2000). *Effective treatments for PTSD: Practice guidelines from the International Society for Traumatic Stress Studies.* New York: Guilford.

Foa, E. B., & Rothbaum, B. O. (1998). *Treating the trauma of rape: Cognitive-behavioral therapy for PTSD.* New York: Guilford.

Franz, D.R., Jahrling, P.B., Friedlander, A.M., McClain, D.J., Hoover, D.L., Bryne, W.R., et al. (1997). Clinical recognition and management of patients exposed to biological warfare agents. *Journal of the American Medical Association, 278,* 399–411.

Friedman, P.D., Saitz, R., Gogineni, A., Zhang, J.X., & Stein, M.D. (2001). Validation of the screening strategy in the NIAAA. Physicians' Guide to Helping Patients with Alcohol Problems. *Journal of Studies on Alcohol, 62,* 234–238.

Gentilello, L. M., Rivara, F. P., Donovan, D. M., Jurkovich, G. J., Daranciang, E., Dunn, et al. (1999). Alcohol interventions in a trauma center as a means of reducing the risk of injury recurrence. *Annals of Surgery, 230,* 473–483.

Goldman, M., Brown, S., & Christiansen, B. (2000). Alcohol Expectancy Questionnaire (AEQ). In Task Force for the Handbook of Psychiatric Measures (Ed.), *Handbook of psychiatric measures* (pp. 476–477). Washington, DC: American Psychiatric Association.

Guskiewicz, K.M., McCrea, M., Marshall S.W., Cantu, R.C., Randolph, C., Barr, W., Onate, J.A., & Kelly, J.P. (2003). Cumulative effects associated with recurrent concussion in collegiate football players: The NCAA concussion study. *JAMA, 290*, 2549–2555.

Jones, F.D. (1995a). Disorders of frustration and loneliness. In F.D. Jones, L.R. Sparacino, V.L. Wilcox, J.M. Rothberg, & J.W. Stokes (Eds.), *War psychiatry* (pp. 63–83). Washington, DC: Borden Institute.

Jones, F.D. (1995b). Psychiatric principles of future warfare. In F.D. Jones, L.R. Sparacino, V.L. Wilcox, J.M. Rothberg, & J.W. Stokes (Eds.), *War psychiatry* (pp. 113–132). Washington, DC: Borden Institute.

Jordan, B. K., Marmar, C. R., Fairbank, J. A., Schlenger, W. E., Kulka, R. A., Hough, R. L., & Weiss, D. S. (1992). Problems in families of male Vietnam veterans with posttraumatic stress disorders. *Journal of Consulting and Clinical Psychology, 60*, 916–926.

Kelly, J.P., Nichols, J.S., Filley, C.M., Lillehie, K.O., Rubinstein, D., & Kleinschmidt-DeMasters, B.K. (1991). Concussion in sports: Guidelines for the prevention of catastrophic outcome. *JAMA, 266*(20), 2867–2869.

King, D.W., King, L.A., & Vogt, D.S. (2003). *Manual for the Deployment Risk and Resilience Inventory (DRRI): A collection of measures for studying deployment-related experiences in military veterans.* Boston, MA: National Center for PTSD.

Kirkland, F. R. (1995). Postcombat reentry. In F. D. Jones, L. Sparacino, V. L. Wilcox, J. M. Rothberg, & J. W. Stokes (Eds.), *War psychiatry* (pp. 291–317). Washington, DC: Office of the Surgeon General.

Koshes, R. J. (1996). The care of those returned: Psychiatric illnesses of war. In R. J. Ursano & A. E. Norwood (Eds.), *Emotional aftermath of the Persian Gulf War: Veterans, families, communities, and nations* (pp. 393–414). Washington, DC: American Psychiatric Press

Kubany, E. S. (1998). Cognitive therapy for trauma-related guilt. In V. M. Follette, J. I. Ruzek, & F. R. Abueg (Eds.), *Cognitive-behavioral therapies for trauma* (pp. 124–161). New York: Guilford.

Kubany, E.S., Abueg, F.R., Owens, J.A., Brennan, J.M., Kaplan, A.S., & Watson, S.B. (1995). Initial examination of a multidimensional model of trauma-related guilt: Applications to combat veterans and battered women. *Journal of Psychopathology and Behavioral Assessment, 17*, 353–376.

Mayorga, M. A. (1997). The pathology of primary blast overpressure injure. *Toxicology. 121* (1): 17–28

Mitchell, J.T., & Everly, G.S. (2000). Critical incident stress management and critical incident stress debriefings: Evolutions, effects and outcomes. In B. Raphael & J.P. Wilson (Eds.), *Psychological debriefing: Theory, practice and evidence* (pp. 71–90). New York: Cambridge University Press.

Najavits, L. M. (2002). *Seeking safety: A treatment manual for PTSD and substance abuse.* New York: Guilford.

Norwood, A. E., Fullerton, C. S., & Hagen, K. P. (1996). Those left behind: Military families. In R. J. Ursano & A. E. Norwood (Eds.), *Emotional aftermath of the Persian Gulf War: Veterans, families, communities, and nations* (pp. 163–196). Washington, DC: American Psychiatric Press.

Proctor, S. P., Heeren, T., White, R. F., Wolfe, J., Borgos, M. S., Davis, J. D., et al. (1998). Health status of Persian Gulf War veterans: Self-reported symptoms, environmental exposures and the effect of stress. *International Journal of Epidemiology, 27,* 1000–1010.

Resick, P. S., & Schnicke, M. K. (2002). *Cognitive processing therapy for rape victims: A treatment manual.* Newbury Park, CA: Sage.

Resnick, H., Acierno, R., Holmes, M., Kilpatrick, D. G., & Jager, N. (1999). Prevention of post-rape psychopathology: Preliminary findings of a controlled acute rape treatment study. *Journal of Anxiety Disorders, 13*

Rothbaum, B. O., Meadows, E. A., Resick, P., & Foy, D. W. (2000). Cognitive-behavioral therapy. In E. B. Foa, T. M. Keane, & M. J. Friedman (Eds.), *Effective treatments for PTSD: Practice guidelines from the International Society for Traumatic Stress Studies* (pp. 60–83). New York: Guilford.

Ruzek, J. I. (2003). Concurrent posttraumatic stress disorder and substance use disorder among veterans: Evidence and treatment issues. In P. Ouimette & P. J. Brown (Eds.), *Trauma and substance abuse: Causes, consequences, and treatment of comorbid disorders* (pp. 191–207). Washington, DC: American Psychological Association.

Ruzek, J. I. & Zatzick, D. F. (2000). Ethical considerations in research participation among acutely injured trauma survivors: An empirical investigation. *General Hospital Psychiatry, 22*

Schlenger, W.E., Caddell, J.M., Ebert, L., Jordan, B.K., Rourke, K.M., Wilson, D., et al. (2002). Psychological reactions to terrorist attacks. Findings from the National Study of Americans' Reactions to September 11. *Journal of the American Medical Association, 288,* 581–588.

Scurfield, R. M., & Tice, S. (1991). Acute psycho-social intervention strategies with medical and psychiatric evacuees of "Operation Desert Storm" and their families. *Operation Desert Storm Clinician Packet.* White River Junction, VT: National Center for PTSD.

Shuster, M.A., Stein, B.D., Jaycox, L.H., Collins, R.L., Marshall, G.N., Elliott, M.N., et al. (2001). A national survey of stress reactions after the September 11, 2001, terrorist attack. *New England Journal of Medicine, 345,* 1507–1512.

Solomon, S., Keane, T., Kaloupek, D., & Newman, E. (1996). Choosing self-report measures and structured interviews. In E. B. Carlson (Ed.), *Trauma research methodology* (pp. 56–81). Lutherville, MD: Sidran Press.

Spielberger, C.D. (1988). *Manual for the State-Trait Anger Expression Inventory.* Odessa, FL: Psychological Assessment Resources.

Steil, R., & Ehlers, A. (2000). Dysfunctional meaning of posttraumatic intrusions in chronic PTSD. *Behaviour Research and Therapy, 38,* 537–558.

Ursano, R.J., McCaughey, B.G., & Fullerton, C.S. (Eds.). (1994). *Individual and community responses to trauma and disaster: The structure of human chaos.* New York: Cambridge University Press.

Vlahov, D., Galea, S., Resnick, H., Boscarino, J.A., Bucuvalas, M., Gold, J., et al. (2002). Increased use of cigarettes, alcohol, and marijuana among Manhattan, New York, residents after the September 11th terrorist attacks. *American Journal of Epidemiology, 155,* 988–996.

Wain, H. J., & Jaccard, J. T. (1996). Psychiatric intervention with medical and surgical patients of war. In R, J. Ursano and A. E. Norwood (Eds.), *Emotional aftermath of the Persian Gulf War: Veterans, families, communities, and nations* (pp. 415–442). Washington, DC: American Psychiatric Press.

Weathers, F.W., Keane, T.M., & Davidson, J.R.T. (2001). Clinician-administered PTSD Scale: A review of the first ten years of research. *Depression and Anxiety, 156,* 132–156.

Wilson, J.P., & Keane, T.M. (Eds.). (1996). *Assessing psychological trauma and PTSD.* New York: Guilford Press.

Wolfe, J. W., Keane, T. M., & Young, B. L. (1996). From soldier to civilian: Acute adjustment patterns of returned Persian Gulf veterans. In R. J. Ursano & A. E. Norwood (Eds.), *Emotional aftermath of the Persian Gulf War: Veterans, families, communities, and nations* (pp. 477–499). Washington, DC: American Psychiatric Press.

Wolfe, J., & Kimerling, R. (1997). Gender issues in the assessment of PTSD. In J. Wilson & T. M. Keane (Eds.), *Assessing psychological trauma and PTSD* (pp. 192–238). New York: Guilford.

Yerkes, S. A., & Holloway, H. C. (1996). War and homecomings: The stressors of war and of returning from war. In R. J. Ursano & A. E. Norwood (Eds.), *Emotional aftermath of the Persian Gulf War: Veterans, families, communities, and nations* (pp. 25–42). Washington, DC: American Psychiatric Press.

Index

About the Authors

Cheryl Lawhorne holds a bachelor's degree in broadcast communications from Virginia Polytechnic Institute and State University. She completed master's degrees in clinical counseling and gerontology from Virginia Tech, as well as postgrad studies in counseling, specializing in post-traumatic stress, combat occupational stress, and traumatic brain injury.

Cheryl is a plankholder for the Wounded Warrior Battalion West at Camp Pendleton, California. She now serves as the deputy program manager for the Recovery Care Coordination Program with the Wounded Warrior Regiment in Quantico, Virginia, under the guidance of Headquarters Marine Corps and the Office of the Secretary of Defense. She was a contributing author to *The Wounded Warrior Handbook* and coauthor of *The Military Marriage Manual*.

Cheryl lives with her sons Evan Alexander and Christian Quinn in Alexandria, Virginia. They are proud to be a United States Marine Corps family.

Don Philpott is editor of *International Homeland Security Journal* and has been writing, reporting, and broadcasting on international events, trouble spots, and major news stories for almost forty years. For twenty years, he was a senior correspondent with Press Association—Reuters, the wire service, and traveled the world on assignments, including Northern Ireland, Lebanon, Israel, South Africa, and Asia.

He writes for magazines and newspapers in the United States and Europe and is a regular contributor to radio and television programs on security and other issues. He is the author of more than ninety books on a wide range of subjects and has had more than five thousand articles printed in publications around the world. His most recent books are *The Workplace Violence Preven-*

tion Handbook, Education Facility Security Handbook, and *Is America Safe?* He is also a coauthor of *The Wounded Warrior Handbook* and *The Military Marriage Manual.* He has written special reports on "Protecting the Athens Olympics," "The Threat from Dirty Bombs," "Anti-Terrorism Measures in the UK," "Nanotechnology and the U.S. Military," and "The Global Impact of the London Bombings."

Born in the United Kingdom, he is now an American citizen working out of Orlando, Florida.